TRENDS IN NEUROIMMUNOLOGY

TRENDS IN NEUROIMMUNOLOGY

Edited by

Maria Giovanna Marrosu
and Carlo Cianchetti
University of Cagliari
Cagliari, Italy
and
Bruno Tavolato
University of Padua
Padua, Italy

PLENUM PRESS • NEW YORK AND LONDON

Library of Congress Cataloging-in-Publication Data

International Symposium on Trends in Neuroimmunology (1988 : Cagliari, Italy)
Trends in neuroimmunology / edited by Maria Giovanna Marrosu and Carlo Cianchetti and Bruno Tavolato.
p. cm.
"Proceedings of an International Symposium on Trends in Neuroimmunology, held September 19-20, 1988, in Cagliari, Italy"--T.p. verso.
Includes bibliographical references.
ISBN 0-306-43510-1
1. Neuroimmunology--Congresses. 2. Central nervous system--Diseases--Immunological aspects--Congresses. I. Marrosu, Maria Giovanna. II. Cianchetti, Carlo. III. Tavolato, Bruno. IV. Title.
[DNLM: 1. Central Nervous System Diseases--immunology--congresses. 2. Neuroimmunomodulation--congresses. WL 300 I625t 1988]
QP355.47.I57 1988
616.8'0479--dc20
DNLM/DLC
for Library of Congress 90-6764
CIP

Proceedings of an International Symposium on Trends in Neuroimmunology, held September 19–20, 1988, in Cagliari, Italy

Printed in the United States of America

PREFACE

Immunology has developed quite impressively over the past decade and perhaps very few fields in medicine or biology have grown so explosively.

Completely new fields have been elucidated in depth. We recall only the definition of the nature and function of HLA antigens at the molecular level, the chemical and functional identification of several cytokines, and the correlation to particular immunological functions of specific epitopes present on cellular membranes.

The extensive application of immunological techniques and concepts to the neurological sciences has led to the development of neuroimmunology, a discipline in its infancy until few years ago. In these last years, neuroimmunology has developed researches in various fields. HLA antigens were studied at the cellular level in brain samples and in CSF cells in several diseases. Cytokines, such as interleukin 1 and 2, gamma- and alpha-interferons, and tumor necrosis factor alpha, were studied at the immunohistological level and with quantitative methods in serum and CSF. With these data, new relevant insights were obtained on the molecular mechanisms underlying CNS immunological diseases. Moreover, neuroimmunological researches were carried on through the development of new and more 'specific' technologies for the study of natural and experimental diseases, the most important of which seem to be, at present, the techniques of cell cultures for cell lines specific to the CNS (oligodendrocytes, astroglia, microglia, meningeal cells, brain capillary cells and tumor cells).

This volume contains contributions presented at the international symposium 'Trends in Neuroimmunology', held at S. Margherita di Pula, Cagliari (Sardinia) from 19-20 September 1988, under the auspices of the International Federation of Multiple Sclerosis Societies. The scientific organization was headed by the Institute of Neuropsichiatria Infantile of the University of Cagliari. Full financial support was given by the Associazione Italiana Assistenza Spastici of Cagliari.

Four main topics were treated in different sessions of the symposium: (1) humoral immunologic studies in CSF, (2) cell studies, (3) immune function of the glia, and (4) CNS diseases and the immune system. This allowed a panoramic view of some of the most promising fields in neuroimmunology. In this respect, the sessions on cell studies and on the immune functions of glia furnished the major contributions in pioneering lines of research. On the other hand, the session on humoral studies demonstrated the vitality of this field, the first one afforded by neuroimmunology, and the last session showed the advanced role of neuroimmunology in some representative clinical problems. The symposium was a really stimulating medium for the discussion of data and for the comparison of different experiences and we hope that this volume may have a similar stimulating role.

We are grateful to the other members of the scientific committee who enthusiastically supported the symposium: Luigi Amaducci (Florence), Mario Battaglia (Trieste), Paolo Livrea (Bari), and Giulio Rosati (Sassari).

We are grateful to Dr Francesco Muntoni, who actively and competently cooperated in the organization of this volume, and to the local staff, Dr Anna Lisa Fratta, Dr Francesco Muntoni, Dr Giovanni Marrosu, Dr Maria Paola Pischedda and Dr Gabriella Spinicci, who all worked very efficiently to ensure the success of the symposium.

Finally, thanks are due to the staff of the Associazione Italiana Assistenza Spastici of Cagliari, which scrupulously took care of the organization of the symposium.

Maria Giovanna Marrosu, MD
Carlo Cianchetti, MD
Bruno Tavolato, MD

CONTENTS

IMMUNE FUNCTIONS OF GLIA

CENTRAL NERVOUS SYSTEM DISEASES AND THE IMMUNE SYSTEM

Humoral Immunologic Studies in Cerebrospinal Fluid

A NEW STRATEGY FOR THE STUDY OF INTRATHECAL IMMUNITY

E. Schüller

Directeur de Recherche (INSERM) Laboratoire
de Neuro-Immunologie, Hôpital de la Salpêtrière,
75651 Paris Cedex 13, France

In its normal state, the central nervous system (CNS) is protected from the circulating immune system. However, each neuro-immunological process can break this sanctuary by two different ways: (1) transudation, a pathological influx of proteins from blood; and (2) intrathecal production of the immune system proteins such as immunoglobulins synthesized by B lymphocytes or complement components by macrophages and probably astrocytes. These two processes can occur either separately or together: the basic question is thus to evaluate the respective contribution of each of these processes when one of these immune proteins is increased in the CSF.

The study of IT immunity has the four following main aims: (1) the definition of the immune pattern; (2) the etiological diagnosis, when possible; (3) the evaluation of the severity; and (4) the monitoring of the course, of the IT process under way.

Our present strategy[1] is outlined in Table 1. Obviously it is necessary to analyze the patient's serum (sampled at the same time as the CSF) using the same immunochemical and microbiological methodologies.

INTRATHECAL SYNTHESIS OF IMMUNOGLOBULINS

The ITS of a given protein can be evaluated by subtracting the physiological filtration and the probable transudation of the protein from its CSF concentration.

Physiological Filtration

The calculation of ITS must take into account the physiological filtration of the protein: this factor can be estimated as the normal upper limit concentration of this protein in the CSF.

Abbreviations: IT = intrathecal, ITS = intrathecal synthesis, EID = electro-immunodiffusion.

Table 1. Study of Intrathecal Immunity

Stages	Technique used	Focus	Aim
Intrathecal synthesis of Immunoglobulins	Immunochemical (EID)	Isotyping of Ig	Definition of the Intrathecal Immune pattern (classification)
Evaluation of anti-body specific activity (ASA)	Conventional serological or Immunochemical titrations	Idiotyping of Ig	Search for specificity of the Intrathecal process
Modifications of complement-components (C1q, C3, C4, C3 proA)	Immunochemical (EID)	Activation of the main and/or the alternative way	Search for Intrathecal Immune complexes formation

Transudation

The formula we proposed[2] with Harvey Sagar, 7 years ago, is based on a very simple empirical postulate: an increase of 40 mg/L from the normal mean of CSF albumin corresponds to a transudation of 1/1000 of the plasma proteins. More difficult was to find the equivalence of transudation for each protein compared to that of albumin.

Our first attempt was the determination of IgG transudation equivalence: we took advantage of the fact that an oligoclonal aspect is a good witness of IgG ITS and we were able to perform our estimation on a very large population (with or without blood-CSF barrier disturbance) which allows us to establish this equivalence to 60. A few months later, we determined Clq in CSF[3] a protein with a molecular weight of 400 KDa. From this study (performed on 104 matched sera and CSF) we could calculate a transudation equivalence of 120, as compared to the value of 40 attributed, *a priori*, to albumin. At this time, the relation between the molecular weight of these three proteins and their transudation equivalence appeared as a simple first order algebraic function of $y = ax + b$ type (Fig. 1). This function was confirmed later by the data obtained for two other immunoglobulins (IgM and IgA) and three other complement components (C3, C4, B factor). The control of each formula is very simple, by the analysis of a large number of patients presenting a more or less important transudation of plasma proteins: if the formula is correct, the observed and the expected values must be the same. In patients with a CSF albumin lower or equal to the normal mean of CSF albumin concentration, the subtraction of the 'maximum physiological filtration' is the only calculation.

Each formula, indeed, must be adapted to each laboratory using the values considered as normal according to the local methodology used.

The normal limits, determined in our laboratory by electroimmunodiffusion, are given in Table 2 together with the equivalence values of transudation for each protein. The formula for the calculation of IT IgG synthesis is given in Table 3.

In Table 4 we compared the data obtained by this formula[4], to the ones established by Link[5] or Tourtellotte[6]. These three formulae are, for the most part, in agreement but it is noticeable that in multiple sclerosis (MS) patients, our formula detects more frequently an IT IgG synthesis. Interestingly enough,

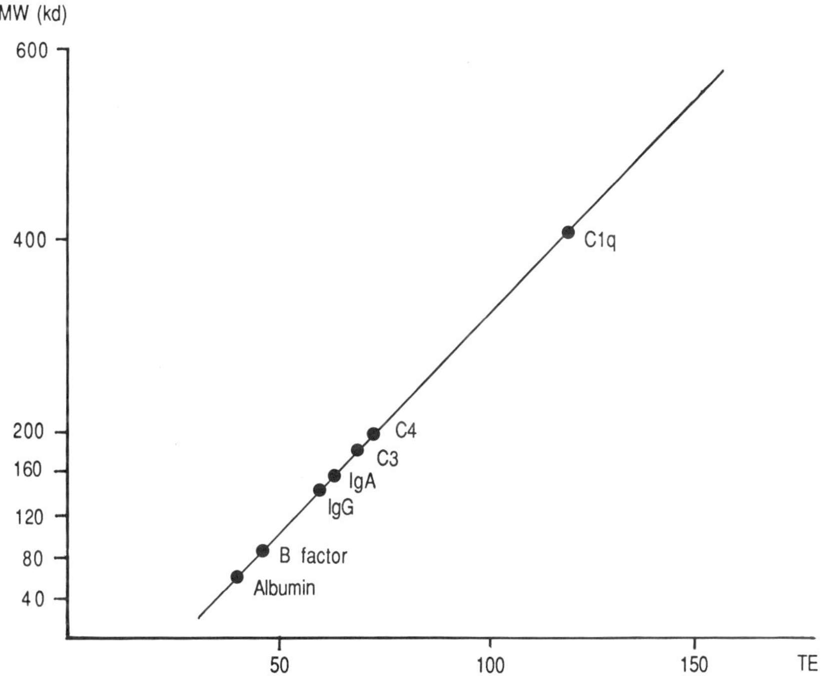

Fig. 1. Molecular weight, in kilodaltons, and transudation equivalence. Transudation equivalence of a protein is calculated as algebraic function ($y = ax + b$), where y is the molecular weight and x the transudation equivalence; a = 4.3 and b = -106. Transudation equivalence values as follows: albumin, 40; B factor, 46; IgG, 60; IgA, 62; C3, 68; C4, 72; C1q, 120; IgM, 246.

Table 2. Molecular Weights, Concentrations, and Transudation Equivalences of Immunity Proteins

	MW (KDa)	Normal Limits (mg/L) Serum	CSF	Transudation equivalences
IgG	150	10000-15000	15-30	60
IgA	160	1000-4000	2-5	62
IgM	960	500-1000	0.2-0.5	246
C1q	400	227-325	0.2-0.5	120
C3	180	700-1138	2-4	68
C4	206	200-400	1-3	72
C3 pro-A	93	72-243	0.2-0.5	46

the number of patients presenting an IT IgG synthesis was found to be significantly similar to the frequency of MS CSF oligoclonal banding ($p < 0.001$).

The intrathecal syntheses given by our formulae are expressed either as an absolute value (in mg/l) or as a percentage of the CSF concentrations: the usefulness of this percentage in calculating antibodies specific activities will be shown later. This first step allows a definition of the CSF immune pattern into four types: normal, transudate (increase of proteins from blood without IT syntheses), inflammatory (ITS without transudation) and meningitis (association of

Table 3. Intrathecal IgG Synthesis (mg/l)

$$\text{CSF IgG} - 30 + \frac{\text{(CSF Alb (mg/l) - CSF Alb n.m.*)}}{60} \text{ (serum IgG) (g/l)}$$

*CSF Alb normal mean = 240 mg/l (by electrophoresis)
or 210 mg/l (by EID)

If CSF albumin is ≤ CSF Alb n.m. = no transudation
In this case: local IgG synthesis = CSF IgG - 30
and if CSF IgG ≤ 30: no local IgG synthesis

Ref: Schuller et Sagar, JNS, 1981, 51:361-370

Table 4. Correlations Between the Three Formulae* of Intrathecal IgG Synthesis

Patients (108)	No ITS† of IgG for F1,F2,F3 (38)	ITS† of IgG for F1,F2,F3 (47)	ITS† of IgG only F2 (23)
Multiple sclerosis (48)	10	25	13
Infectious dis. (22)	3	15	4
Degenerative dis. (21)	20	1	0
Malignant process (5)	2	1	2
Inflammatory dis. (4)	0	3	1
Peripheral neurop. (8)	3	2	3

Conclusion: 79% of the results are in concordance
* F1 = Link, F2 = Schuller and Sagar, F3 = Tourtellotte.
† ITS = Intrathecal synthesis

Table 5. Intrathecal Immunoglobulins Syntheses: Frequencies (%)

	IgG	IgA	IgM
MS (168)	86	7	17
Neurosyphilis* (36)	92	22	61
AIDS (38)	89	42	37

* Positive CSF TPHA.

Statistics:			
	ITS IgM	MS-Neurosyph.	$p < 0.001$
		MS-AIDS	$p < 0.01$
		AIDS-Neurosyph.	$p < 0.05$
	ITS IgA	MS-Neurosyph.	$p < 0.01$
		MS-AIDS	$p < 0.001$

transudation and ITS). Table 5 shows the frequencies of the immunoglobulins ITS: obviously IgG ITS is very common, but the frequencies of IgA and IgM ITS are significantly different in neurosyphilis, AIDS and MS.

The usefulness of ITS determination in the evaluation of the severity and the monitoring of the course of a disease are clearly illustrated by the following two examples: (1) in MS: where a significant correlation (Table 6) can be established between the ITS of IgG and the type of the course, or the disability grade; (2) in Guillain-Barré syndrome: the IgG ITS is significantly linked to the clinical stage, the severity of the process and its duration (Fig. 2). But one of the major

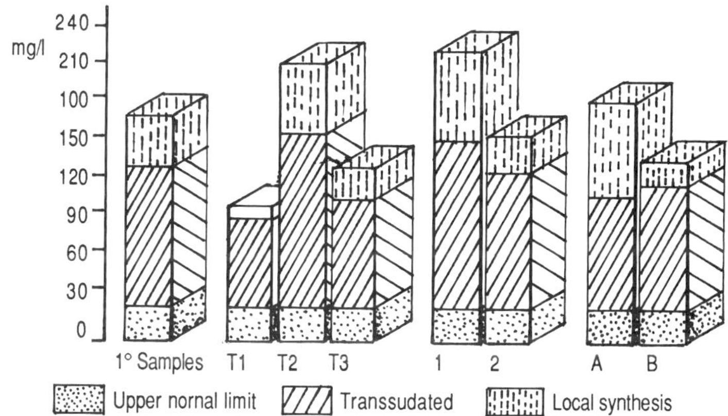

Fig. 2. Guillain-Barré syndrome: course of CSF IgG. LP: first lumbar punction, T1: progression, T2: stabilization of paralysis, T3: regression, 1: severe forms (CNS involvement), 2: middle forms, A: duration > 3 months, B: duration < 3 months.

Table 6. Intrathecal IgG Synthesis, Course, and Disability Degree in 191 MS Patients

Clinical data	Criteria	IgG ITS* (mean ± SE)	Significance (p)
Course	relapsing (116)	40 ± 4.1	< 0.02
	progressive (75)	60 ± 6.8	
Disability (Kurtzke scale)	K1 + K2 (65)	34 ± 5.4	< 0.02 between K1 + K2 and the two other groups
	K3 + K4 (70)	53 ± 5.7	
	K5 - K9 (56)	58 + 8.3	

* ITS = Intrathecal synthesis.

interests of this calculation is certainly the evaluation of the intrathecal antibody specific activity.

INTRATHECAL ANTIBODY SPECIFIC ACTIVITY (IT ASA)

When the same antibody is identified in the serum and the CSF two questions must be solved: (1) Is the specific immunity detected in the CSF the result of a filtration or of a pathological transudation of the antibody present in the blood? (2) If an ITS of this antibody can be established, is the activity of B lymphocytes in the CNS similar or higher than in the circulating blood?

ASA is the ratio between the antibody activity (expressed in arbitrary units) and the concentration of the corresponding immunoglobulin (in mg/l):

The antibody activity is defined as the serological titre. Thus,

$$ASA = \frac{\text{serological titre}}{[\text{Ig}]\ (\text{mg/l})}$$

For convenience, this ASA is expressed in units of 10^{-3}. If a CSF ASA is higher than the corresponding serum ASA, an ITS of the antibody is obvious.

By definition, CSF ASA is:

$$\left[\begin{array}{c} \text{Serum ASA} \\ \text{x} \\ \text{percentage of CSF IgG} \\ \text{of plasmatic origin} \end{array} \right] + \left[\begin{array}{c} \text{IT ASA} \\ \text{x} \\ \text{percentage of IgG} \\ \text{IT produced} \end{array} \right]$$

Thus:

$$\text{IT ASA} = \frac{\text{CSF ASA - (serum ASA x percentage of IgG from serum)}}{\text{percentage of IT IgG}}$$

From this calculation three possibilities can be found:

(1) no ITS of the antibody which is of plasmatic origin only;
(2) an IT ASA equal or inferior to the corresponding ASA in serum. This signals a general immune response not related to an IT stimulus; or
(3) an IT ASA higher (2 to 1000 times) than the corresponding serum ASA, suggesting an IT antigenic stimulation greater than in the other parts of the body.

An example of this calculation is given in Table 7, demonstrating that a very common antibody titre in the CSF can be the sign of a strong intrathecal immune response.

Results indicated in Table 8 show that in three infectious CNS diseases (syphilis, AIDS and SSPE) IT ASA is clearly higher than the corresponding serum ASA. In MS, anti-measles IT ASA is significantly higher than serum ASA, and the rubella IT ASA/serum ASA ratio is also very high. In contrast herpes ratio is much lower. As previously published[9] no significant difference can be established between SSPE and MS patients concerning anti-measles IT ASA, a fact suggesting a strong intrathecal antigenic stimulation in both diseases. Another fact is given by anti-herpes IT ASA in AIDS patients: in 8/20 patients investigated this IT ASA was higher than the anti-herpes ASA in serum, suggesting a possible replication of herpes virus inside the CNS of these patients[10]. A similar mode of calculation has been proposed in neuro syphilis by Prange[11] and for CSF IgM, by Muller[12].

Table 7. Intrathecal Antimeasles Antibody Specific Activity (ASA) in a MS Patient

	Serum	CSF	IT synthesis
IgG (mg/l)	12000	100	50 mg/l (50%)
Measles antibodies (serological titre)	60	2	
ASA	60/12000 = 5*	2/100 = 20*	

CSF ASA is 4 times higher than serum ASA

Thus: $\text{Intrathecal ASA} = \frac{20 - (0.5 \times 5)}{0.5} = 35$

Conclusion: IT ASA is 7 times higher than serum ASA

* Units: 10^{-3}

Table 8. Serum and Intrathecal ASA in Neurosyphilis, AIDS, SSPE and MS

Disease	Test	Serum ASA (mean ± SE)	Intrathecal ASA (mean ± SE)	IT ASA / Serum ASA
Neurosyphilis (21)	TPHA	2101 ± 783	28591 ± 6835	14
AIDS (38)	Elavia	400 ± 121	7042 ± 1829	18
SSPE (32)	Measles HIA	24 ± 6	172 ± 45	7
.(82)	Measles HIA	11 ± 1	100 ± 22	9
MS .(49)	Rubella HIA	16 ± 2	95 ± 17	6
.(16)	Herpes HT	17 ± 3	42 ± 16	2.5

INTRATHECAL VARIATIONS OF THE COMPLEMENT

Each of the four complement components can be intrathecally synthesized, and the rate of these syntheses can be calculated using the appropriate formulae. In a certain number of patients an abnormal depletion of these components can be observed. This depletion is calculated from the lower limit value of this component concentration in the normal CSF.

As indicated in Table 9, this negative result is expressed as a percentage with reference to the expected concentration.

The frequencies of these different IT activations of complement in neuro syphilis, AIDS, SSPE and MS are given in Table 10.

In the Guillain-Barré syndrome[8], the depletion of C3 is significantly linked to the IT IgG synthesis. In neurosyphilis the depletion of C3 is correlated to IT IgM synthesis. Conversely C4 depletion seems very rare, but IT C4 synthesis is relatively frequent, particularly in AIDS patients[10]. In these latter patients, the demonstration of IT C4 synthesis is probably a good marker of macrophages activity inside the CNS. Finally, the study of these intrathecal complement activations may be an index of the activity of the current intrathecal process and, consequently, of its evolutivity. However this calculation implies the transudation of the corresponding proteins: in our present experience it can be performed only if an intrathecal immunoglobulin synthesis is established, a fact suggesting the transudation of molecules with a similar molecular weight.

Table 9. C3 Intrathecal Depletion

$$\text{CSF C3 (mg/l)} - \left[2 + \frac{\text{CSF Alb} - 240}{68} (\text{serum C3 (g/l)})\right]$$

The negative result is expressed in percentage with reference to the expected concentration

Examples: $5 - \left[2 + \frac{640 - 240}{68} (0.8)\right] = -1.7$ mg/L

Expected concentration: 6.7 mg/l

This negative value of -1.7 mg/L corresponds to a depletion of

$$\frac{-1.7 \times 100}{6.7} = -25\%$$

Table 10. Intrathecal Activation of Complement Components: in Neurosyphilis, AIDS, SSPE and MS

Disease	C 3		C 4		B factor	
	ITS*	ITD*	ITS	ITD	ITS	ITD
Neurosyphilis* (21)	1 (5%)	13 (62%)	10 (48%)	2 (10%)	8 (38%)	1 (5%)
AIDS† (38)	4 (11%)	11 (29%)	29 (76%)	2 (5%)	-	-
SSPE (18)	2 (11%)	2 (11%)	5 (28%)	1 (6%)	-	-
MS (140)	12 (9%)	52 (37%)	18 (13%)	5 (4%)	27 (19%)	2 (1%)

* CSF TPHA serology positive, † Serum HIV1 serology positive, ITS = Intrathecal synthesis, ITD = Intrathecal depletion.

Table 11. NOM: CALD..., Age: 1920, Date: 10/4/85, Diagnostic: méningo encèphalite herpétique - 6e jour
Proteines totales du L.C.R. 2,70 G/L

DOSAGE	SERUM		L.C.R.		INTRATHECAL	
	mg/l	%	mg/l	%	synthese consomma	%
Electrophorese:						
Prealbumine		1	81	3		
Albumine eph		49	1701	63		
A1		5	162	6		
A2		16	135	5		
B1		8	135	5		
B2		4	81	3		
G		17	405	15		
Prealbumine E.I.D.	-					
Albumine E.I.D.	-		-			
Type dosage			EPH			
Albumine pour calcul			1701			
IgA	2700		12.5			
IgG	12200		350		22,93	7
IgM	540		10,4		6,69	64
CRP	0		0			
C3	1160		12,8		-14,12	-52,0
C43	530		7,4		-4,35	-37,0
C3 proA	260		4		-4,46	-52,0

ANTICORPS	SERUM		L.C.R.		INTRATH.
	Titre	A.S.A.	Titre	A.S.A.	A.S.A.
PNA	261	107	6	86	0
Herpes	40	3	16	46	617

CONCLUSIONS

The study of the intrathecal immunity, initiated 45 years ago by Kabat[13] and followed later by the introduction of CSF electrophoresis (demonstrating the oligoclonal aspect[14-15]), is now more sophisticated. All its parameters can be calculated very precisely by a computer using a special logical. The example given in Table 11 illustrates clearly the interest of these analyses in a herpes-encephalitis patient at Day 6. If our present conclusions are accepted, an intrathecal viral stimulus is very probable in MS patients, more or less cross-reactive with measles antigens. In AIDS patients an intrathecal replication of viruses other than HIV-1 can be also suspected. These two points in addition to many others, in our opinion, justify further research in this direction.

ACKNOWLEDGEMENTS

This research was supported by Institut National de la Santé et de la Recherche Médicale (INSERM) and Association pour la Recherche sur la Sclérose en Plaques (ARSEP). We thank B. Zalc for his help in English translation, and M. Josien for statistics and personal assistance.

REFERENCES

1. E. Schuller, L'analyse de l'immunité intrathecale, *Presse Med.* 17:155-160 (1988).
2. E. Schuller and H. Sagar, Local synthesis of CSF immunoglobulins: a neuroimmunological classification, *J.Neurol.Sci.*, 51:261-370 (1981).
3. E. Schuller and M. Helary, Determination in the nanogram range of C1q in serum and unconcentrated CSF by electro-immunodiffusion, *J.Immunol.Meth.*, 56:159-165 (1983).
4. E. Schuller, S. Benabdallah, H.J. Sagar, J. Reboul, and L. Tömpe, IgG synthesis within the central nervous system, *Arch.Neurol.*, 44, 600-604 (1987).
5. G. Tibbling, H. Link, and S. Ohman, Principles of albumin and IgG analyses in neurological disorders. I- Establishment of reference values, *Scand.J.Clin.Lab.Invest.*, 37:385-390 (1977).
6. W. W. Tourtellotte, On cerebrospinal fluid immunoglobulin G (IgG) quotients in multiple sclerosis and other diseases. A review and a new formula to estimate the amount of IgG synthesized per day by the central nervous system, *J.Neurol.Sci.*, 10:279-304 (1970).
7. E. Schuller and H.J. Sagar, Central nervous system IgG synthesis in multiple sclerosis. Application of a new formula, *Acta Neurol.Scand.*, 67:365-371 (1983).
8. P. Amarenco, B. Sauron, E. Schuller, F. Chain, and P. Castaigne, Serum and CSF humoral immunity in Guillain-Barré syndrome: clinical correlations, *J.Neurol.Sci.*, 80:129-142 (1987).
9. E. Schuller, B. Allinquant, P. Lebon, H.J. Sagar, A. Govaerts, and J.D. Degos, Measles specific antibody activity in serum and locally synthesized CSF IgG fractions: results in SSPE, MS, and other neurological diseases, *in:* "Subacute sclerosing panencephalitis: a reappraisal", F. Bergamini, C.A. Defanti, P. Ferrante, eds, Elsevier Sci. Pub. BV, pp.293-304 (1986).
10. J. Reboul, E. Schuller, G. Pialoux, M.A. Rey, P. Lebon, B. Allinquant, and F. Brun-Vezinet, Intrathecal immunity in 37 patients seropositive for anti-HIV1 antibody, *J.Neuro.Immunol.*, 16:156 (1987).
11. H. W. Prange, M. Moskophidis, H.L.I. Schipper, and F. Muller, Relationship between neurological features and intrathecal synthesis of IgG antibodies to treponema pallidum in untreated and treated human neurosyphilis, *J.Neurol.*, 230:241-252 (1983).
12. F. Muller, M. Moskophidis, and H. W. Prange, Demonstration of locally synthesized immunoglobulin M antibodies to treponema pallidum in the central nervous system of patients with untreated neurosyphilis, *J.Neuroimmunol.*, 7:43-54 (1984/85).
13. E. A. Kabat, D. H. Moore, and H. Landow, An electrophoretic study of the protein components in cerebro-spinal fluid and their relationship to the serum proteins, *J.Clin.Invest.*, 21:571-577 (1942).

14. A Löwenthal, M. Van Sande, and D. Karcher, The differential diagnosis of neurological diseases by fractionating electrophoretically the CSE-gamma-globulins, *J.Neurochem.*, 6:51-56 (1960).
15. E. C. Laterre, A. Callewaert, J. F. Heremans, and Z. Sfaello, Electrophoretic morphology of gamma-globulins in cerebrospinal fluid of multiple sclerosis and other diseases of the nervous system, *J.Neurol.*, 20:982-990 (1970).

IMMUNOLOGICAL FINDINGS IN THE CSF OF HIV-1 INFECTED PATIENTS

A. De Rossi, P. Gallo*, A. Amadori, M.G. Piccinno*, A. Del Mistro, S. Pagni*, M.L. Calabrò, L. Chieco-Bianchi, and B. Tavolato*

Institute of Oncology, Interuniversity Center for Research on Cancer, and
*Institute of Neurology, University of Padova, School of Medicine, Padova, Italy

INTRODUCTION

Both peripheral and central nervous system disorders have been described in patients with the acquired immunodeficiency syndrome (AIDS).[1-8] Increasing evidence indicates that the human immunodeficiency virus type 1 (HIV-1) is neurotropic and infects the nervous system early in the course of systemic virus spread.[9-14] Ultrastructural and hybridization analyses of brain tissue from AIDS patients have revealed that HIV-1 replication occurs predominantly in cells of macrophage/microglial lineage.[15-16] However, the relationship between the neurological/psychiatric symptoms associated with HIV-1 infections of the central nervous system (CNS) and the HIV-1-induced immunological abnormalities at the cellular level is still unclear.

In the present study, we analyzed intrathecal synthesis of anti-HIV 1 antibodies (HIV-1 Ab) and viral antigens in 45 HIV-1 infected patients. In addition, CSF and serum levels of interleukin-2 (IL-2), soluble IL-2 receptors (sIL-2R) and tumor necrosis factor alpha (TNFα) were evaluated.

MATERIALS AND METHODS

Patients

A group of 45 HIV-1-seropositive patients forms the basis of this study. All were Italians from the Veneto region (northeast Italy). The patients were classified as asymptomatic (9), or affected by AIDS-related complex (ARC) (6) and AIDS (30). Twelve were female, and 33 were male. Thirty-five subjects were intravenous drug abusers, four were homosexuals, two were haemophiliacs, one was a blood recipient, one had sexual activity in an endemic area, and one was a child born to an HIV-1 seropositive mother; in two cases the risk factor was not identified.

Cryptococcal meningitis was the most frequent neurologic complication (nine cases), followed by cerebral toxoplasmosis (six cases) and aseptic meningitis (two cases). Only one patient showed clinical signs of AIDS-dementia complex, i.e., mental slowing with impaired memory and concentration, apathy, loss of spontaneity, and social withdrawal; a computerized tomographic (CT) scan disclosed severe, diffuse cortical atrophy with ventricular dilatation, and attenuation of the white matter.

Routine CSF Studies

These were performed as previously described in detail.[17-18] Briefly, CSF was obtained by atraumatic lumbar puncture, and cell counts were performed within 30 min. Albumin and IgG levels in undiluted CSF and in corresponding serum were determined by immunoprecipitation nephelometry. The CSF-serum albumin ratio assessed the blood-brain barrier (BBB) integrity;[19] given the age range of our patients values higher than 5.5 were considered the expression of BBB damage. The IgG index (equal to CSF/serum IgG : CSF/serum albumin) evaluated intrathecal IgG synthesis quantitatively,[19] and values higher than 0.7 were considered positive.

To demonstrate IgG oligoclonal band patterns in undiluted CSF, a very sensitive method was used[20] with previously described modifications.[17] Briefly, agarose isoelectric focusing (AIEF) was followed by protein transfer to nitrocellulose membrane (BA 85, 45 μm, Schleicher and Schuell, Kassel, West Germany), double immunofixation (primary antibody, rabbit anti-human IgG (Fc); second antibody, mouse biotinylated anti-rabbit IgG), avidin-biotin amplification, and peroxidase staining (Vectastain ABC Kit, PK 4001, Vector Laboratories, Inc., Burlinghame, CA). Two or more IgG bands seen in CSF at pH values above 7.0 (in addition to those seen in corresponding serum run in parallel) were considered to represent oligoclonal IgG bands.

Affinity-driven Transfer of Focused IgG

To detect virus-specific oligoclonal IgG in undiluted CSF, affinity-driven transfer of focused IgG by capillary attraction was performed[21] with the minor modification previously described.[13] Briefly, nitrocellulose membranes (BA 85, 45 μm, Schleicher and Schuell) were cut into sheets measuring 50 x 100 mm, and coted with 0.5 mg of HIV viral lysate (Litton Bionetics, Charleston, SC) by overnight incubation at room temperature. Membrane saturation was controlled by incubating a nitrocellulose fragment for 1 hr with anti-p 15 anti-p 24 monoclonal antibodies (de Pont de Nemours, Wilmington, DE) at 1:100 final dilution. The immunoreaction was detected by incubation for 1 hr with peroxidase-linked anti-mouse IgG (Vector) followed by 4-chloro-1-napthol as peroxidase substrate.

After AIEF of paired CSF and serum specimens, the antigen-coated nitrocellulose membrane was placed on top of the gel and then covered by several sheets of moistened filter paper, a glass plate, and a 200 g weight to support affinity-driven transfer of IgG. After 1 hr at room temperature, affinity-blotted IgG bands were detected either by the avidin-biotin-peroxidase stain described above, or by a protein A-gold stain followed by silver enhancement (BioRad, Richmond, CA). The latter method was used to avoid the background that usually appears when antigen-coated nitrocellulose membranes are developed with the avidin-biotin system.

Paired CSF and serum samples from patients with multiple sclerosis, neurosyphilis, herpes simplex encephalitis, and post-infectious encephalomyelitis, with very prominent CSF oligoclonal IgG bands, were used as controls to ensure affinity transfer specificity.

Absorption of Virus Antibodies

As previously described,[22] serum aliquots and undiluted CSF specimens were adjusted to the same IgG concentration, mixed with virus antigens, and incubated for 30 min at 37°C, and then for 2 hr at 4°C. After high-speed centrifugation (20,000 x g), the supernatants were studied by isoelectric focusing and IgG immunofixation as described above.

Enzyme-linked Immunoadsorbent Assay

Enzyme linked immunoadsorbent assay (ELISA) was carried out in serum and CSF as previously described.[23,24] Briefly 100 μl of 1:20 diluted serum or 100 μl of undiluted CSF were added to 5 μg/ml HIV-1 lysate virus-coated 96-well microtiter plates and incubated overnight at 4°C. After 1 hr incubation at room temperature with peroxidase-linked anti-human IgG (Kirkegaard & Perry Laboratories, Gaithersburg, MD), orthophenylenediamine substrate was added and the plates were read on a MCC Titertek Multiscan apparatus (Flow Laboratories, Irvine, UK).

Western Blot Assay

The Western blot (WB) assay was performed in serum, CSF, and supernatant (SN) of lymphocyte cultures (see below) as reported elsewhere.[25,26] Briefly, nitrocellulose strips with HIV-1 viral proteins were incubated overnight at room temperature with serum, CSF, or SN, at 1:100, 1:50, and 1:4 final dilutions, respectively. Each strip was incubated for 1 hr with 1 x 10^6 CPM of affinity-purified ^{125}I-labeled goat anti-human IgG and then mounted and placed against X-ray film. Commercial WB kits (du Pont, BioRad) were also employed in a set of experiments, with minor modifications of the manufacturer's instructions.

Serum, CSF, and lymphocyte culture SN of the same patient were tested within the same experiment.

HIV Antigen Determination in Serum and in CSF

The search for viral antigens in serum and CSF was accomplished by using the HIV-1 p24 ELISA system (de Pont), according to the manufacturer's instructions.

Virus Detection

Peripheral blood lymphocytes (PBL) from individual patients were purified by Ficoll-Plaque (Pharmacia, Uppsala, Sweden), as previously described,[27] and cultured at 1 x 10^6 cells/ml in RPMI medium in the presence of 1 μg/ml phytohemagglutinin (PHA-P, Difco, Detroit, MI) at 37°C for 48 hr. Cells were then washed, and cultured in RPMI containing 10% T cell growth factor (Cellular Products, Inc., Buffalo, NY) and 1000 U/ml anti alpha-interferon (Miles Scientific, Naperville,).

The CSF were filtered through a 0.22 μm Millipore filter (Millipore, Bedford, MA); 1 ml was inoculated into normal PBL that had been treated for 48 hr with PHA-P, and the cultures were carried out as described above.

Aliquots (1 ml) of the culture SNs were collected every 3-4 days for reverse transcriptase (RT) assay, and complete medium was replaced. RT assay was performed as previously described[28] and results were expressed as mean CPM [^{3}H]-thymidine incorporation in each assay performed in duplicate. Positive and negative controls were constituted by cell-free SN from HIV-1-infected and non-infected PBL cultures, respectively. SN showing a [^{3}H]-thymidine uptake three times greater than values obtained in negative controls were scored as positive.

In Vitro Antibody Production

The procedure to evaluate *in vitro* anti-HIV-1 specific antibody production has been described in detail elsewhere.[14,29] Briefly, PBL were cultured at 1 x 10^6 cells per ml in 24-well culture plates (Costar, Cambridge, MA). CSF lymphocytes (CSFL) were obtained by low-speed centrifugation of 30 ml of CSF, and were cultured at concentrations ranging from 5 x 10^4 to 3 x 10^5 cells per ml in 96-well microtiter plates (Costar).

Both PBL and CSFL were cultured in the presence of pokeweed mitogen (PWM, Gibco, Grand Island, NY) at a 1:100 final dilution. SN from PBL and CSFL cultures were collected after 7 and 14 days of culture, respectively, centrifuged, and tested for HIV antibodies by WB analysis.

TNF Alpha Bioassay and ELISA

The TNF-sensitive L-M cell line (murine connective tissue fibroblast) was obtained from the American Type Culture Collection. A serum-free bioassay was carried out on as previously described.[30] Human recombinant TNF-α and neutralizing rabbit anti-human TNF-α antisera were purchased from Genzyme Corporation (Boston, MA). Data are given as percent (%) survival ratio or units of TNFα, where 1 unit/mL (U/mL) is defined as the concentration that produces lysis of 50% of the L-M cells.

The commercially available ELISA kit for TNFα quantitation (Byokine, T Cell Sciences, Cambridge, MA) was used with minor modifications. TNFα levels in CSF and sera were quantified by ELISA since the bioassay gave false positive results when testing patient's sera. In our hands, 20 pg/mL of TNFα corresponded to 1 U/mL.

IL-2 and sIL-2R ELISA

IL-2 enzyme immunoassay was performed as previously reported[31] by using an ELISA method (Intertest 2, Genzyme Co, Boston, MA) that allows detection of as little as 0.04 U/ml of IL-2.

sIL-2-R levels were determined by the commercial sandwich enzyme immunoassay Cell-free (T-cell Sciences, Cambridge, MA), according to the manufacturer's instructions.

RESULTS

HIV-1 Antibodies in Serum, CSF and Lymphocyte SN

CSF data for all the patients included in the study are shown in Table 1.

BBB damage was demonstrated in 23 patients (four asymptomatic, two ARC, 17 AIDS). These included the 17 cases with neurologic complications, and six others who had no evidence of neurologic disease at the time of sampling. Increased IgG index and IgG oligoclonal bands were demonstrated in 24 and 16 patients respectively, while an IgG oligoclonal pattern was found in both CSF and serum in eight patients.

Affinity-driven transfer and virus antibody absorption studies disclosed that the oligoclonal IgG patterns were partly recognized by HIV-1 Ag (Fig. 1). Some bands were not recognized, and were interpreted as an expression of polyclonal B cell activation or antibodies against opportunistic agents.

All but four patients had detectable levels of HIV-1 Ab in CSF. The HIV-1 Ab patterns were little influenced by the state of BBB permeability.

In asymptomatic and ARC patients, the HIV-1 Ab profile in CSF was usually more complete compared to patients with AIDS. Interestingly, the CSF pattern in 18 cases did not show anti-p24 reactivity, which was instead detected in the respective sera.

Table 1. CSF Data of the 45 HIV-1-infected Patients Included in the Study

HIV-1 infected patients 45	Alb $\frac{CSF}{SERUM}$ ratio ($N \leq 5.5$)	IgG Index ($N \leq 0.7$)	Oligoclonal IgG bands +	HIV-1 Ab* +	HIV-1 Ag* +	Pleiocytosis† +	IL-2 +	sIL-2R +	TNFα +
Asymptomatic 9	4/9	5/9	5/9	8/9	0/9	1/9	nd	nd	0/9
ARC 6	2/6	2/6	2/6	6/6	1/6	1/6	nd	nd	0/6
AIDS 30	17/30	17/30	9/30	27/30	6/30	17/30	0/30	12/30	0/30
	23/45 (51%)	24/45 (53%)	16/45 (35.5%)	41/45 (91%)	7/45 (15.5%)	19/45 (42%)	0/30 (0%)	12/30 (40%)	0/45 (0%)

* HIV-1 antibodies (HIV-1 Ab) and HIV-1 antigens (HIV-1 Ag)
† Pleiocytosis indicates more than 3 white-cells per mm^3 in the CSF
nd = Not done

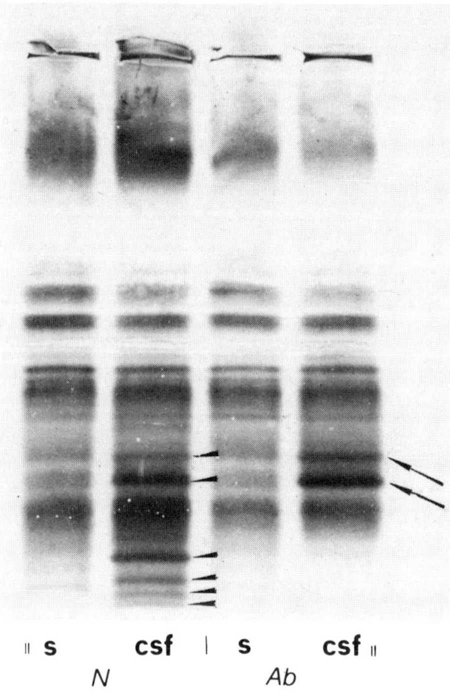

Fig. 1. Paired serum and cerebrospinal fluid (CSF) sample from a WR6 patient. N=Native specimens; Ab=specimens after absorption of HIV-1 antibodies. In native CSF a clear pattern of oligoclonal IgG is visible (arrowheads). After absorption, the oligoclonal pattern partly disappeared, indicating that at least some IgG bands were anti-HIV-1 antibodies. However, two quite prominent IgG bands (arrows) were not recognized by HIV-1 antigens. Since the patient had cryptococcal meningitis at the moment of lumbar puncture, these bands may be anti-cryptoccocus antibodies or an expression of a polyclonal B-cell activation.

All SN from PBL and CSFL cultures showed HIV-1 Ab on WB assay. SN from CSFL cultures however showed reactivity only against *env* products, while SN from PBL cultures showed broader ranges of specificities.

HIV-1 Antigen Detection and Virus Isolation

Specific p24 *gag* protein was detected in seven CSF examined. RT activity was found in four SN of cultures obtained by infection of normal PBL with cell-free CSF.

Cytokine Detection

IL-2 and TNFα were evaluated in 30 cases, and were never detected in CSF nor in serum. Increased sIL-2R levels (exceeding the range of values observed in control subjects) were found in 27 out of 30 sera (Fig. 3). The mean value was significantly higher (mean $\pm$ SD = 685 $\pm$ 146) than in the normal control group (mean $\pm$ SD = 158 $\pm$ 56, $p < 0.001$), and was quite similar to figures reported in HIV-1-infected patients.[32,33] Detectable levels of sIL-2R were also found in 12 CSF which also presented increased white cell counts (eight cryptococcal meningitis, two cerebral toxoplasmosis, two 'aseptic' meningitis).

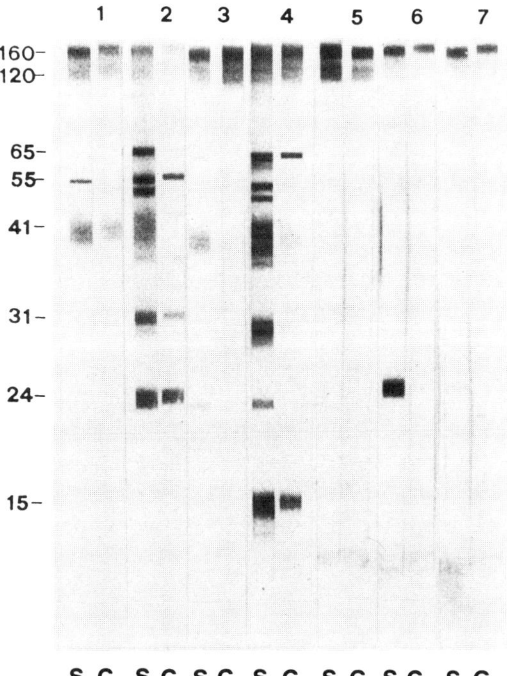

Fig. 2. Representative patterns of HIV-1 antibodies in Western Blot analysis of paired serum (S) and CSF (C) samples from seven different patients.

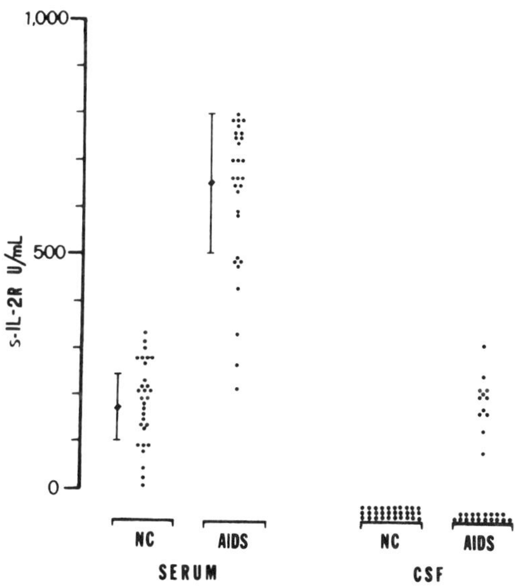

Fig. 3. Serum and CSF soluble interleukin-2 receptor (sIL-2R) levels in patients with AIDS and in non-risk controls (normal controls = NC).

DISCUSSION

Almost all the patients in this study had intrathecal synthesis of anti-HIV-1 Ab in the CSF. In addition, virus was detected in seven CSF. As previously reported,[13] we noticed that the presence of BBB damage was not sufficient to modify the anti-HIV-1 Ab pattern in the CSF.

The detection of IgG bands with anti-HIV-1 specificities, and the frequent increase in the IgG index (50% of the cases), as well as the finding of '*in vitro*' anti-HIV-1 Ab production by CSFL in patients with no neurological complication and different degrees of immunodeficiency all indicate a very early CNS infection by HIV-1.

A comparison of CSF and serum HIV-1 Ab profiles detected by WB analysis disclosed some interesting differences. Most CSF had no anti-core specificity, while the majority of the sera had both anti-core and anti-*env* antibodies. The absence of anti-*gag* antibodies in CSF could represent a different and more rapid evolution of HIV-1 infection in the CNS. However, a segregation of antibody-producing cells within the CNS, probably due to a different expression of viral proteins, should also be considered. These findings further emphasize that CNS involvement in HIV-1 patients occurs frequently and at very early stages of viral spread throughout the body.

TNFα, a cytokine produced by activated macrophages[34] is produced by activated microglial cells,[35] and is able to produce demyelination '*in vitro*'. Since HIV-1 replication in the brain seems to occur predominantly in cells of macrophage/microglia lineage, we tested the hypothesis that an abnormal production of TNFα by infected microglial cells could account for the diffuse demyelination very often seen in such patients.

A TNF-like activity was never detected in CSF or serum of the HIV-1 patients in this study, even when diffuse myelin damage was well documented by CT or MRI. Hence, TNFα does not seem to play a role in HIV-1 induced CNS demyelination. Nevertheless, intracerebral production of TNFα followed by its complete absorption at the target tissue level cannot be excluded.

Increased levels of sIL-2R have already been described in both CSF and serum of AIDS patients.[31,32,36] However, the mechanism(s) accounting for the increased sIL-2R production, and the subsequent pathophysiological implications have not yet been clarified. We found increased titers of sIL-2R in almost all sera studied, while IL-2 was never detected. Moreover, detectable sIL-2R levels were found in 12 CSF specimens, and were invariably associated with an increased number of white cells. The discrepancy between sIL-2R and IL-2 levels in both serum and CSF of HIV-1 patients suggests that the mechanism underlying the abnormal sIL-2R production does not necessarily involve IL-2 synthesis by T-cells.

Studies on CSF soluble mediators of the immune response will be useful in elucidating the early events that take place within the CNS during HIV-1 infection.

ACKNOWLEDGEMENTS

This work was supported by grants from Consiglio Nazionale delle Ricerche, Progetto Finalizzato 'Oncologia', Associazione Italiana per le Ricerche sul Cancro, Ministero della Pubblica Instruzione, and from the Veneto Region. The authors gratefully acknowledge the invaluable assistance of Ms P. Segato and Ms A. Leone in the preparation of this manuscript.

REFERENCES

1. Various Authors, Retroviruses in the Nervous System, Proceedings of a Symposium sponsored by the N.I.H. Bethesda, MD, May 4-6, 1987, *Ann.Neurol.*Vol. 23 (suppl.) (1988).
2. J. R. Berger, The neurological complications of HIV infection, *Acta Neurol.Scand.*77 (suppl. 116):40-76 (1988).
3. B. A. Navia, B. D. Jordan, and R. W. Price, The AIDS dementia complex: I. Clinical features, *Ann.Neurol.*, 19:517-524 (1986).
4. B. A. Navia, E. S. Cho, C. K. Petito, and R. W. Price, The AIDS dementia complex II, Neuropathology, *Ann.Neurol.*, 19:525-535 (1986).
5. C. K. Petito, B. A. Navia, E. S. Cho et al., Vacuolar myelopathy pathologically resembling subacute combined degeneration in patients with acquired immunodeficiency syndrome (AIDS), *N.Engl.J.Med.*, 312:874-879 (1985).
6. W. D. Snider, D. M. Simpson, S. Nielsen et al., Neurological complication of acquired immune deficiency syndrome: analysis of 50 patients, *Ann.Neurol.*, 14:403-418 (1983).
7. D. D. Ho., M. G. Sargadmaran, L. Resnick et al., Primary human T-lymphotropic virus type III infection, *Ann.Intern.Med.*, 103:880-883 (1985).
8. M. C. Dalakas, G. H. Pezeshkpour, M. Gravell et al., Polymyositis associated with AIDS retrovirus, *JAMA*, 256:2381-2383 (1986).
9. D. D. Ho., T. R. Rota, R. T. Schooley et al., Isolation of HTLV-III from cerebrospinal fluid and brain tissue of patients with neurologic syndromes related to the acquired immunodeficiency syndrome, *N.Engl.J.Med.*, 313:1493-1497 (1987).
10. G. M. Show, H. E. Harper, B. H. Hahn et al., HTLV III infection in brains of children and adults with AIDS encephalopathy, *Science*, 227:177-182 (1987).
11. F. Chiodi, A. Sönnerborg, J. Albert et al., Human immunodeficiency virus infection of the brain. I. Virus isolation and detection of HIV specific antibodies in the cerebrospinal fluid of patients with varying clinical conditions, *J.Neurol.Sci.*, 85:245-257 (1988).
12. L. Resnick, F. Di Marzo-Veronese, J. Schupbach et al., Intra BBB-synthesis of HTLV-III specific IgG in patients with neurologic symptoms associated with AIDS or AIDS-related complex, *N.England.J.Med.*, 313:1498-1504 (1985).
13. P. Gallo, A. De Rossi, A. Amadori et al., Central Nervous System involvement in HIV infection, *AIDS Res.Hum.Retroviruses*, 4:211-221 (1988).
14. A. Amadori, A. De Rossi, P. Gallo et al., Cerebrospinal fluid lymphocytes from HIV-I infected patients synthesize HIV-specific antibody *in vitro*, *J.Neuroimmunol.*, 18:181-186 (1988).
15. S. Koenig, H. E. Gendelman, J. M. Orenstein et al., Detection of AIDS virus in macrophages in brain tissue from AIDS patients with encephalopathy, *Science*, 233:1089-1093 (1986).
16. C. A. Wiley, R. D. Schrier, J. A. Nelson et al., Cellular localization of human immunodeficiency virus infection within the brains of acquired immunodeficiency syndrome patients, *Proc.Natl.Acad.Sci. USA*, 83:7089-7093 (1986).
17. P. Gallo, F. Bracco, L. Battistin, and B. Tavolato, Detection of IgG oligoclonal bands in unconcentrated CSF by means of agarose isoelectric focusing, double immunofixation, peroxidase staining, and avidin-biotin amplification, *Ital.J.Neurol.Sci.*, 6:275-282 (1985).
18. P. Gallo, F. Bracco, and B. Tavolato, Blood-brain barrier damage restricts the reliability of quantitative formulae and isoelectric focusing in detecting intrathecally synthesized IgG, *J.Neurol.Sci.*, 84:87-93 (1988).
19. G. Tibbling, H. Link, and S. Ohman, Principles of albumin and IgG analysis in neurological disorders. I. Establishment of reference values, *Scand.J.Clin.Lab.Invest.*, 37:385-390 (1977).

20. T. Olsson, V. Kostulas, and H. Link, Improved detection of oligoclonal IgG in cerebrospinal fluids by isoelectric focusing in agarose, double immunofixation staining and avidin-biotin amplification, *Clin.Chem.*, 30:1246-1249 (1984).
21. R. Dorries and V. Ter Meulen, Detection and identification of virus-specific oligoclonal IgG in unconcentrated cerebrospinal fluid by immunoblot technique, *J.Neuroimmunol.*, 7:77-89 (1984).
22. F. Vartdal and B. Vandvik, Multiple Sclerosis, Electrophocused "bands" of oligoclonal CSF IgG do not carry antibody activity against Measles, Varicella Zooster, or Rotaviruses, *J.Neurol.Sci.*, 54:99-107 (1982).
23. W. C. Saxinger and R. C. Gallo, Application of the indirect enzyme-linked immunosorbent assay microtest to the detection and surveillance of human T cell leukemia-lymphoma virus, *Lab.Invest.*, 49:371-377 (1983).
24. A. De Rossi, P. Gallo, B. Tavolato et al., Search for HTLV-I and LAV/HTLV-III antibodies in serum and CSF of multiple sclerosis patients, *Acta Neurol.Scand.*, 74:161-164 (1986).
25. J. Schupbach, M. Popovic, R. V. Gilden et al., Serological analysis of a subgroup of human T-lymphotropic retroviruses (HTLV-III) associated with AIDS, *Science*, 224:503-505 (1984).
26. A. De Rossi, O. Dalla Gassa, A. Del Mistro et al., HTLV III and HTLV I-infection in populations at risk in the Veneto region of Italy, *Eur.J.Cancer Clin.Oncol.*, 22:411-418 (1986).
27. A. Amadori, G. Faulkner-Valle, A. De Rossi et al., HIV-mediated immunodepression: *in vitro* inhibition of T-lymphocyte proliferative response by ultraviolet-inactivated virus, *Clin.Immunol.Immunopathol.*, 46:37-54 (1988).
28. H. M. Rho and R. C. Gallo, Biochemical and immunological properties of the DNA polymerase and RNAse-H activities of purified feline leukemia virus reverse transcriptase, *Cancer Lett.*, 10:207-221 (1980).
29. A. Amadori, A. De Rossi, G. Faulkner-Valle, and L. Chieco-Bianchi, Spontaneous *in vitro* production of virus-specific antibodies by lymphocytes from HIV-infected subjects, *Clin.Immunol.Immunopathol.*, 46:342-351 (1988).
30. S. M. Kramer and M. E. Carver, Serum-free bioassay for the detection of tumor necrosis factor, *J.Immunol.Meth.*, 93:201-206 (1986).
31. P. Gallo, M. Piccinno, S. Pagni, and B. Tavolato, Interleukin-2 levels in serum and CSF of multiple sclerosis patients, *Ann.Neurol.*, 24:795-797 (1988).
32. G. Pizzolo, F. Vinante, A. Sinicco et al., Increased levels of soluble interleukin-2 receptor in the serum of patients with human immunodeficiency virus infection, *Diag.Clin.Immunol.*, 5:180-183 (1987).
33. B. E. Kloster, P. A. John, L. E. Miller et al., Soluble interleukin-2 receptors are elevated in patients with AIDS or at risk of developing AIDS, *Clin.Immunol.Immunopathol.*, 45:440-446 (1987).
34. L. J. Old, Tumor Necrosis Factor (TNF), *Science*, 230:630-632.
35. K. Frei, C. Siepl, P. Groscuth et al., antigen presentation and tumor cytotoxicity by interferon-gamma treated microglial cells, *Eur.J.Immunol.*, 17:1271-1278 (1987).
36. K. K. Sethi and H. Näher, Elevated titers of cell-free interleukin-2 receptor in serum and cerebrospinal fluid specimens of patients with acquired immunodeficiency syndrome, *Immunol.Lett.*, 13:179-184 (1986).

DISEASE DURATION, RELAPSE RATE AND CLINICAL COURSE IN MULTIPLE SCLEROSIS: RELATION TO IgG PRODUCTION WITHIN THE BLOOD BRAIN BARRIER

Paolo Livrea, Maria Trojano, Isabella Laura Simone, Carlo Avolio, Francesca De Robertis, Brigida Coluccia, Cecilia Manzari, and Antonio Rosato

Institute of Nervous and Mental Disease,
University of Bari, I-70124 Bari, Italy

The interrelationships between the cerebrospinal fluid (CSF) abnormalities and the clinical course of multiple sclerosis (MS) have been investigated in several studies. Clinical variables are often difficult to define in MS, and some of them (age, disease duration, number of bouts, disability) are likely to be interdependent.[2] Moreover, the lack of uniformity in the definition of clinical and temporal parameters employed in the assessment of the disease course[10] hampered comparable results in different studies.

The mononuclear CSF pleocytosis seemed to be more frequent during MS clinical exacerbations,[24] while it appeared to decline along with the increasing disease duration.[23] The presence of an intra blood-brain barrier (BBB) synthesis of oligoclonal IgG in the majority of patients has been known for a long time.[33] The sensitivity of the separation methods accounts for the discrepancies about the prevalence, as well as the predictive negative or positive values of this finding.[9] Quantitative measures of the synthesis do not correlate clearly with the presence or the number of the abnormal IgG CSF fractions and appear likely to be influenced by the BBB permeability properties and by the CSF dynamics also.[17] Nevertheless, MS lesions have been confirmed by autoptic examination in cases without CSF IgG abnormality,[4] and a benign clinical course seems to be associated to the normal IgG pattern.[29] No agreement exists about the temporal invariance of the IgG pattern during the disease course, because a stability,[36] a decrease or an increase[31] in the pattern complexity have been reported during sequential CSF samples obtained in individual patients over wide ranges of time intervals. The amount of intra BBB produced IgG correlated in some series to the entity of CSF pleocytosis;[32] by means of CSF studies performed in strictly controlled clinical conditions an increased IgG synthesis has been demonstrated during exacerbations,[14] but cultured CSF mononuclear cells appeared to produce higher IgG amounts along with the duration of remissions.[22] The BBB opening to serum proteins is usually slight and confined to few patients, without clear correlations with other CSF abnormalities or clinical variables;[34] information about the BBB selectivity properties at the lesion sites are few[1] and only the progressive course of the disease seems to be characterized by a BBB selectivity loss to large serum proteins.[30]

This report details a further investigation on the interrelationships between the CSF IgG abnormalities and the clinical course of MS. The results indicate that the intra BBB IgG response, the CSF pleocytosis and the BBB permselectivity

Table 1. Diagnosis, Disease Phase and Therapy in MS Patients at CSF Examination

	Phase			Corticosteroids†		
	Active	Inactive	Progressive	Never given	Discontinued*	Yes
Clinically definite	18	5	9	10	14	8
Probable initial latent	28	5	=	11	10	12
Progressive probable	=	=	16	16	=	=
Progressive possible	=	=	10	10	=	=
Suspected	6	3	=	9	=	=
Total	52	13	35	56	24	20

† Decadron 8 mg/daily for 1-15 days, tapered in 30-60 days
* from 1-36 months.

also, show dynamic, interrelated changes consistent with the different phases and the course of the disease.

MATERIALS AND METHODS

Patients

One hundred MS patients were rated according to the clinical confidence of the diagnosis,[20] the history of previous corticosteroid treatment, the disability (EDSS),[11] number of bouts, phase, course[2 8] and duration of the disease (Tables 1 and 2). The retrospective analysis of the clinical history was recorded by means of a standard questionnaire structured with closed questions and answers, and assuming precise temporal limits[28] in the definition of the disease events. The reliability of the questionnaire was evaluated by the agreement (unweighted K statistic)[6] of two independent raters assessing the history of the patients on the same day and after one month. The agreement was high (K in the range 0.35-0.9; z in the range 3.2-9.8) for all the examined items.[16]

Methods

The count of CSF mononuclear cells, the assay of CSF IgG index,[15] the analysis of abnormal IgG fractions in CSF isoelectric spectrotype,[18] the assessment of the BBB permselectivity to serum albumin (CSF/serum albumin x 10^3) and alpha$_2$macroglobulin (CSF alpha$_2$macroglobulin index = CSF/serum alpha$_2$macroglobulin : CSF/serum albumin)[17] were determined in all MS patients. The values obtained in age and sex matched neurological patients affected by disorders presumably not associated with CSF abnormalities (vascular headache, idiopathic partial epilepsy, dizziness), were considered as controls, and their mean + 2SD was assumed as the upper normal limit (Table 3).

Statistical Analysis

Student t test, chi square, and multiple regression were used. The multiple regressions among all CSF (mononuclear cells/µl, CSF IgG index, CSF/serum albumin x 10^3, CSF alpha$_2$macroglobulin index, number of abnormal IgG fractions in the CSF isoelectric spectrotype) and clinical (age, disease duration, disability,

Table 2. Age, Disease Duration (months), Bouts and Disability (mean ± SD) in MS Patients.

		Age	Disease duration	No. of bouts	Disability
Clinically definite	(32)	34 ± 9	104 ± 72	3.7 ± 1.5	3.1 ± 1.1
Probable initial latent	(33)	27 ± 10	15 ± 27	1.9± 1.3	2.8 ± 1.3
Suspected	(16)	25 ± 11	6 ± 10	1	1 ± 0.7
Progressive probable	(10)	43 ± 14	109 ± 101	=	4 ± 1.9
Progressive possible	(9)	43 ± 13	65 ± 73	=	2 ± 0.7

Table 3. CSF Mononuclear Cells, Amount of Intra BBB IgG Synthesis, BBB Permselectivity to Albumin and Alpha$_2$Macroglobulin, Number of Abnormal IgG Fractions in CSF Isoelectric Spectrotype (mean ± SD) in Controls and MS Patients

	Controls (No.31)	MS Patients(No.100)		%
CSF mononuclear cells/µl	1 ± 0.5	4.7 ± 2.4	*	50%
CSF IgG index	0.45 ± 0.08	0.94 ± 0.54	*	72%
CSF/serum albumin x 10^3	3.7 ± 1.4	4.7 ± 2.4	*	13%
CSF alpha$_2$macroglobulin index	0.21 ± 0.07	0.29 ± 0.15	*	22%
No. of abnormal CSF IgG fractions	0	10.6 ± 7.2		100%

% = Frequency of abnormal values in MS patients; * = Student *t* test $p < 0.01$.

number of bouts) variables were separately tested in the following groups: clinically definite MS (N=32); probable initial or latent MS (N=33); progressive probable MS (N=16); progressive possible MS (N=10); suspected MS (N=9); primary progressive (N=26); secondary progressive (N=9); primary and secondary progressive (N=35); active phase of exacerbation (N=52); clinically definite in active phase (N=18); probable initial or latent in active phase (N=28); active phase in patients never treated (N=28) or treated (N=20) by corticosteroids; first bout in never treated patients (N=14); and stationary disease (N=13). Significant partial correlations between variables were determined by the *t* values of the respective partial regression coefficients. Only significant *t* values are reported in the Tables.

RESULTS

The frequency of the abnormal CSF values found in MS patients is reported in Table 3. The number of CSF mononuclear cells, the BBB permeability to serum albumin and the number of abnormal IgG fractions in CSF spectrotype appeared to change in relation to the phase of the disease. The lack of CSF pleocytosis and an abnormal BBB permeability to serum albumin characterized the chronic progression of the disease. Patients with clinical inactivity had low number of abnormal IgG fractions in the CSF isoelectric spectrotype, compared to patients suffering from an acute exacerbation or a chronic progression of the disease (Table 4).

By keeping constant all CSF and clinical parameters, the amount of intra BBB IgG synthesis correlated in every group with the number of the abnormal IgG fractions in the CSF isoelectric spectrotype. In some groups with a relapsing

Table 4. CSF Parameters During Different Phases of MS Clinical Course

	Active	Inactive	Progressive
No. of patients	52	13	35
CSF mononuclear cells/μl	10.7 ± 17	8.9 ± 16	3.9 ± 3.8 *
CSF IgG index	0.93 ± 0.49	0.76 ± 0.48	0.94 ± 0.52
CSF/serum albumin x 10^3	4.52 ± 2.3	4.31 ± 1.2	5.1 ± 2.8 *
CSF alpha2macroglobulin index	0.27 ± 0.15	0.3 ± 0.2	0.29 ± 0.15
No. of abnormal CSF IgG fractions	10.1 ± 7.9	5.2 ± 2.6 *	10.3 ± 6.4

* = Chi square, $p < 0.001$.

Table 5. Multiple Correlations Among CSF Parameters in MS Significant Partial Regression t Values

Disease phase, diagnosis (No. of patients)	IgG index vs No. of abnormal IgG fractions	IgG index vs No. of mononuclear cells	No. of mononuclear cells vs No. of abnormal IgG fractions
Active, all patients (52)	7.58 [a]		
Active, no steroids (28)	5.38 [a]	2.58 [c]	
Active, definite (18)	4.93 [a]		
Active, probable initial (28)	6.53 [a]	3.15 [c]	-2.33 [d]
Progressive, all patients (35)	5.81 [a]		
Inactive, all patients (13)	2.27 [d]		
Definite (32)	3.97 [a]		-2.21 [d]
Probable initial (33)	6.65 [a]	2.9 [b]	-2.07 [d]
Primary progressive (26)	5.94 [a]		

a = $p < 0.001$; b = $p < 0.02$; c = $p < 0.01$; d = $p < 0.05$
The number of patients is given in parentheses.

remitting course and an active phase of the disease, the amount of the intrathecal IgG synthesis and the amount of the CSF mononuclear cells also correlated. Nevertheless, by keeping constant all CSF and clinical parameters, the number of mononuclear cells had a negative correlation with the complexity of the CSF IgG isoelectric spectrotype in both clinically definite and probable initial latent disease. During an untreated active phase of the disease this relationship seemed to emerge more clearly (Table 5).

The number of bouts and the duration of the disease both accounted for the variability of the number of the abnormal IgG fractions in the CSF isoelectric spectrotype and for the amount of the intra BBB synthesis as well. In patients with active relapsing remitting disease, as the number of previous bouts increased, the number of abnormal CSF IgG fractions increased too, while the amount of intra BBB IgG synthesis decreased. In such patients, the number of bouts had a significant partial regression coefficient with the disease duration, (t=5.33, $p < 0.005$), but this parameter appeared to be negligible for the quantitative changes of the intrathecal IgG synthesis. In patients who suffered more than one bout (clinically definite or probable initial latent disease), at a constant bout number, the disease duration and the amount of the intra BBB synthesis correlated (Table 6).

In patients with either primary or secondary chronic progression of symptoms from the disease onset, a longer disease duration appeared to be accompanied by an increased number of abnormal IgG fractions in the CSF isoelectric spectrotype, together with a decline of the overall amount of the intra BBB IgG synthesis (Table 6).

No correlation was found between the CSF IgG abnormalities and the BBB permselectivity to serum proteins. In patients with active disease the correlation between BBB permeability to albumin and age was retained. However, during both active and stationary disease, the BBB permeability to albumin correlated to

Table 6. Multiple Correlations Among CSF and Clinical Parameters in MS Significant Partial Regression *t* Values

Disease phase, diagnosis		No. of abnormal IgG fractions	No. of bouts vs IgG index	No. of bouts vs No. of abnormal IgG fractions	Duration vs IgG index
Active, all patients	(52)	2.48 [c]	-2.52 [c]		
Active, definite	(18)	2.45 [c]			2.94 [c]
Active, probable initial	(28)				2.18 [d]
Progressive, all patients	(35)			3.19 [a]	-2.26 [d]
Primary progressive	(26)			3.14 [b]	-2.22 [d]

a = $p < 0.005$; b = $p < 0.01$; c = $p < 0.02$; d = $p < 0.05$
The number of patients is given in parentheses.

Table 7. Multiple Correlations Between BBB Permselectivity, CSF Pleocytosis and Clinical Parameters in MS Significant Partial Regression *t* Values

Disease phase, diagnosis		CSF/serum albumin x 1000 vs age	CSF/serum albumin x 1000 vs No. of bouts	CSF alpha$_2$macroglobulin index vs CSF mononuclear pleocytosis
Active, all patients	(52)	2.1 [a]	2.1 [a]	
Active, clinically definite	(18)	2.1 [a]		2.12 [a]
Stationary, all patients	(11)		2.66 [a]	
Clinically defomote	(32)			2.17 [a]
Probable initial latent	(33)		2.07 [a]	

a = $p < 0.05$
The number of patients is given in parentheses.

the number of previous bouts. In active clinically definite disease, the entity of CSF pleocytosis correlated to the entity of BBB permselectivity to alpha$_2$-macroglobulin (Table 7).

DISCUSSION

Dynamic changes in the amount and in the heterogeneity of the IgG production, interrelated with the CSF pleocytosis, occur within the BBB during the different types of MS clinical course. All these parameters, together with the BBB permselectivity, appear to be influenced by the duration and the activity of the disease.

The relapsing remitting course of the disease is characterized by: (1) an amount of intra BBB IgG synthesis influenced by the disease duration and by the occurrence of new bouts; (2) a complexity of CSF IgG isoelectric spectrotype related to the number of bouts; (3) CSF pleocytosis displaying opposite correlations with the amount and the isoelectric spectrotype complexity of the intra BBB IgG synthesis respectively; and (4) a damage of BBB permselectivity related to the mononuclear pleocytosis and to the occurrence of new bouts.

The positive correlation between CSF pleocytosis and the IgG synthesis has already been found.[32] Changes in CSF IgG pattern obtained in patients with optic neuritis, later developing typical MS symptoms,[27] are consistent with the low amounts and the restricted isoelectric heterogeneity of the IgG synthesis at the early stages of the disease. Both CSF pleocytosis and IgG synthesis increase until new bouts develop, thereafter they seem to decline, with an additional complexity of the CSF IgG isoelectric spectrotype, and a slight, partially irreversible, opening of the BBB to serum proteins.

Quantitative CSF IgG changes, with high synthesis rate during the exacerbations of the disease, have already been detected in sequential studies covering one remission and one relapse in the same patients.[14] The decline of the intra BBB IgG synthesis following new bouts could be consistent with the reduced IgG amount produced by cultured cells in response to pokeweed mitogen within 3 weeks after an attack[22] and with the high density of T suppressor cells found at the edge of old plaques.[35]

Changes in the CSF IgG pattern during the course of the disease are still debated;[31,36] differences in patient selection and in the IgG separation methods likely explain the discrepancies of the results. In our hands, the simultaneous analysis of sequential CSF samples obtained in 17 relapsing remitting MS patients after intervals of 0.5-8 years indicated that the complexity of CSF IgG isoelectric spectrotype was unchanged in eight patients, increased in four and decreased in five. The CSF/serum ratio did not differ significantly in each patient and the duration of CSF storage did not influence the isoelectric IgG pattern. No clinical parameter (severity of the clinical course, phase and spatial dissemination of the disease) accounted for this elusive result.

Many events could be reflected by the change of CSF IgG isoelectric pattern. The appearance of new and/or the intermittent activation of preexisting B cell clones has been demonstrated during the disease course;[27] nevertheless, although the molecular basis and the functional significance of the IgG isoelectric spectra in health and disease are unknown, the discrete fractions separated according to the pI do not represent individual antibodies,[5,13] and the content of oligosaccarides or syaloglycopeptides seems mainly to account for their heterogeneity.[33] The occurrence of relapses, with the formation of new lesions or with a new activity in the preexisting lesions, could be accompanied either by an activation of new B cell clones, or changes in enzymatic activities at myelin membranes,[26] vascular endothelium and leucocytes,[19] or both, and could induce an enrichment of the abnormal fractions in the CSF isoelectric spectrum.

The BBB opening which accompanies the disease activity seems to be characterized by two different phenomena: a reversible loss of selectivity for the large serum proteins, significantly depending on the mononuclear pleocytosis; and a partially stable increase in permeability to small serum proteins, persisting after the occurrence of new bouts. CT[3] and NMR[21] imaging support the BBB permeability changes during the disease course. Moreover, bioptic studies of MS lesions suggest that the increased number of pinocytotic vesicles at endothelia, rather than the opening of tight junctions, accounts for the increased protein transfer through the CNS microvasculature.[1] Experimental models of allergic encephalomyelitis[12] indicate that mononuclear cells go through endothelial junctions: according to the CSF data, these large temporary openings likely favour the disproportionate passage of large serum proteins along with the mononuclear infiltration. The increase in endothelial permeability to serum albumin seems to be not necessarily connected to the tight junction dynamics. An increased number of pinocytotic vesicles can maintain a proportional passage of serum proteins irrespective of their size, assuming that the vesicle size does not increase,[17] so as indicated by morphometric studies of MS lesions.[1] The activity of lesions with clinically recordable symptoms seems to be followed by such an event. The activity of astrocytes may be a source of differentiation signals for several aspects of endothelial barrier, but its role in pinocytotic regulation is not elucidated.[8]

It is well known that most of MS patients suffer a secondary chronic disability progression after years of relapsing remitting symptoms.[2] Subclinical relapsing remitting disease activity has been postulated to occur before the development of primary progressive forms.[7] It is worthwhile noting that the CSF changes reflecting the occurrence of additional bouts appear to be similar to the CSF abnormalities which characterize the primary progressive course. In fact, low CSF mononuclear cells, high BBB permeability to albumin, decline in the intra BBB IgG synthesis rate and increase in CSF IgG isoelectric heterogeneity set up after long lasting relapsing remitting course and are also found during the primary chronic progression.

Further analysis of a larger series and sequential studies in individual patients with rigorously defined clinical and paraclinical[25] follow up are necessary to confirm the prognostic value of these CSF parameters. The changes in immune function which occur within BBB during the MS course could be used in patients who have a disability progression and/or a relapse rate of uncertain prognosis[37] and could be related to the different response of the disease variables (number and severity of bouts; development of chronic progression) to the immunosuppressive treatments.

ACKNOWLEDGEMENTS

The skilful technical assistance of Mr Umberto Minerva, Mr Giuseppe Salamanno, Mrs Silvia Casciaro and Mr Salvatore Perrone is gratefully acknowledged. This work was supported by grants of CNR (N.87.00340.56), MPI (40%) and AISM.

REFERENCES

1. W. J. Brown, The capillaries in acute and subacute multiple sclerosis plaques: A morphometric analysis, *Neurology*, 28:84-92 (1978).
2. C. Confraveaux, G. Aimard, and M. Devic, Course and prognosis of multiple sclerosis assessed by the computerized data processing of 349 patients, *Brain*, 103:281-300 (1980).
3. G. C. Ebers, F. V. Vinuela, T. Feasby, and B. Bass, Multifocal CT enhancement in multiple sclerosis, *Neurology*, 34:275-280 (1980).

4. M. A. Farrell, J. C. E. Kaufmann, J. J. Gilbert, J. H. Noseworthy, M. A. Amstrong, and G. C. Ebers, Oligoclonal bands in multiple sclerosis: clinical, pathologic correlations, Neurology, 35:212-218 (1985).
5. K. Felgenhauer and H. Mohrman, Evaluation of immunoglobulin diversity, *In:* Electrophoresis 81, R.C. Allen and P. Arnaud, eds, De Gruyter, Berlin, pp 427-432 (1981).
6 J. L. Fleiss, Statistical methods for rate and proportions, Wiley, New York (1973).
7. T. Fog and F. Linnemann, The course of multiple sclerosis in 73 cases with computer designed curves, *Acta Neurol.Scand.*, 46, supp 47, 1-175 (1970).
8. G. W. Goldstein, Endothelial cell-astrocyte interactions. A cellular model of the blood-brain barrier, *Ann NY Acad.Sci.*, 529:31-39 (1988).
9. V. K. Kostulas, H. Link, and A. K. Lefvert, Oligoclonal IgG bands in CSF. Principles for demonstration and interpretation based on findings in 1114 patients, *Arch.Neurol.*, 44:1041-1044 (1987).
10. J. F. Kurtzke, Multiple sclerosis: What's in a name? *Neurology*, 38:309-316 (1988).
11. J. F. Kurtzke, Rating neurologic impairment in multiple sclerosis: An expanded disability status scale (EDSS), *Neurology*, 33:1444-1452 (1983).
12. P. Lampert and S. Carpenter, Electron microscopic studies on the vascular permeability and the mechanism of demyelination in experimental acute encephalomyelitis, *J.Neuropathol.Exp.Neurol.*, 26: 11-24 (1965).
13. A. R. Latner, T. Marshall, and M. Gambie, Microheterogeneity of serum myeloma immunoglobulins revealed by a technique of high resolution two-dimensional electrophoresis, *Electrophoresis*, 1:82-89 (1980).
14. H. Link, CSF immunoglobulins and clinical course, *In:* "Multiple Sclerosis Research in Europe', O. R. Hommes, ed., MTP Press, Lancaster, pp 231-239 (1986).
15. H. Link and G. Tibbling, Principles of albumin and IgG analyses in neurological disorders, III, evaluation of IgG synthesis within the central nervous system in multiple sclerosis, *Scand.J.Clin.Lab.Invest.*, 37:397-401 (1977).
16. P. Livrea, M. Trojano, C. Avolio, F. De Robertis, C. Manzari, G. C. Logroscino, and A. Rosato, Reliability of a structured interview with closed questions for assessment of multiple sclerosis (MS) clinical course, *In:* "International MS Converence, Abstract Book", p VI/9 (1988).
17. P. Livrea, M. Trojano, I. L. Simone, G. B. Zimatore, L. Pisicchio, G. C. Logroscino, and G. Cibelli, Heterogeneus models for blood-cerebrospinal fluid barrier permeability to serum proteins in normal and abnormal cerebrospinal fluid/serum protein concentration gradients, *J.Neurol.Sci.*, 64:245-258 (1984).
18. P. Livrea, M. Trojano, I. L. Simone, G. B. Zimatore, G. Lamontanara, and R. Leante, Intrathecal IgG synthesis in multiple sclerosis, Comparison between isoelectric focusing and quantitative estimation of CSF IgG, *J.Neurol.*, 224:159-169 (1981).
19. J. Lospalluto, K. Fehr, and M. Ziff, Degradation of immunoglobulins by intracellular proteases in the range of neutral pH, *J.Immunol.*, 105:886-897 (1970).
20. W. I. MacDonald and A. M. Halliday, Diagnosis and classification of multiple sclerosis, *Brit.Med.Bull.*, 33:4-8 (1977).
21. D. H. Miller, P. Rudgr, G. Johnson, B.E. Kendall, D. G. Macmamus, I. F. Moseley, D. Barns, and W. I. McDonald, Serial gadolinum enhanced magnetic resonance imaging in multiple sclerosis, *Brain*, 3:927-939 (1988).
22. J. Oger and M. O'Gorman, Changes in immune function in multiple sclerosis are associated with clinical activity in both relapsing and progressive disease, *Neurology*, 38: supp 1, 238-239 (1988).

23. J. E. Olsson, H. Link, and R. Muller, Immunoglobulins abnormalities in multiple sclerosis. Relations to clinical parameters: diability, duration and age of onset, *J.Neurol.Sci.*, 27:233-245 (1976).
24. J. E. Olsson and H. Link, Immunoglobulins abnormalities in multiple sclerosis. Relations to clinical parameters: exacerbations and remissions, *Arch.Neurol.*, 28:392-399 (1973).
25. C. M. Poser, D. W. Paty, L. Sheinberg, W. I. McDonald, F. A. Davis, G. C. Ebers, K. P. Johnson, W. A. Sibley, D. H. Silberberg, and W. W. Tourtellotte, New diagnostic criteria for multiple sclerosis. Guidelines for research protocols, *Ann.Neurol.*, 13:227-231 (1983).
26. M. Saito and K. Yur, Further characterization of a myelin associated neuroaminidase: Properties and substrate specifity, *J.Neurochem.*, 47:632-641 (1986).
27. M. Sandberg-Wollheim, B. Vandvik, and E. Norby, The intrathecal immune response in the early stage of multiple sclerosis, *J.Neurol.Sci.*, 81:45-53 (1987).
28. G. A. Shumacher, G. Beebe, and R. F. Kiblett, Problems of experimental trials of therapy in multiple sclerosis: report by the Panel of the Evaluation of Experimental trials of Therapy in Multiple Sclerosis, *Ann.NY.Acad.Sci.*, 122:552-568 (1965).
29. L. Stendahl-Brodin and H. Link, Relation between benign course of multiple sclerosis and low grade humoral immune response in cerebrospinal fluid, *J.Neurol.Neurosurg.Psychiat.*, 43:102-105 (1980).
30. T. Takeota, Y. Shinohara, K. Furumi, and K. Mori, Impairment of blood-cerebrospinal fluid barrier in multiple sclerosis, *J.Neurochem* , 41:1102-1108 (1983).
31. E. J. Thompson, P. Kaufmann, and P. Rudge, Sequential changes in oligoclonal pattern during the course of multiple sclerosis, *J.Neurol.Neurosurg.Psychiat.*, 46:115-118 (1983).
32. E. J. Thompson, L. M. Luxon, J. Jethwa, R. C. Shortman, and Paule, On the relationship of CSF pleyocitosis to immunoglobulin levels as estimated by different techniques, *J.Neuroimmunol.*, 2:321-330 (1982).
33. W. W. Tourtellotte, The cerebrospinal fluid in multiple sclerosis, *In:* "Handbook of Clinical Neurology", vol 47, P.J. Vinken, G.W. Brujn and H.L. Klawans, eds, Elsevier, Amsterdam, pp 79-130 (1985).
34. W. W. Tourtellotte and B. I. Ma, Multiple sclerosis: The blood-brain barrier and the measurements of de novo central nervous system IgG synthesis, *Ncurology.*, 28:76-83 (1978).
35. V. Traugott, E. L. Reinherz, and C. S. Raine, Multiple sclerosis. Distribution of T cells subsets, and Ia positive macrophages in lesions of different ages, *J.Neuroimmunol.*, 4:201-221 (1983).
36. M. J. Walsh and W. W. Tourtellotte, Temporal invariance and clonal uniformity of brain and cerebrospinal fluid IgG, IgA and IgM in multiple sclerosis, J.Exp.Med., 163:41-53 (1986).
37. B. G. Weishenker and G. C. Ebers, The natural history of multiple sclerosis, *Can.J.Neurol.Sci.*, 14:255-261 (1987).

ON THE INTRATHECAL SYNTHESIS OF IMMUNOGLOBULINS: DETECTION OF BSF-2/IL-6 IN CSF

P. Gallo, K. Frei, D. Leppert and A. Fontana

Section of Clinical Immunology, Departments of Neurology and Neurosurgery, University Hospital of Zürich, Zürich, Switzerland

INTRODUCTION

Increased Ig indexes and oligoclonal IgG bands in the cerebrospinal fluid (CSF) are commonly found in multiple sclerosis (MS) as well as in other inflammatory diseases of the central nervous system (CNS) (ie, neurosyphilis, subacute sclerosing panencephalitis (SSPE), post-infectious encephalomyelitis, Lime's disease).[1-9] The mechanisms underlying the intrathecal synthesis of immunoglobulins are not yet well understood. In MS, the segregation within the CNS of B-cell clones, primed during exposure to a variety of exogenous antigens, and then activated in the brain by a polyclonal B-cell activator, has been suggested.[10] In the present report we have investigated CSF samples for the presence of B-cell activating cytokines. One such factor, Interleukin-6 (IL-6) was detected in the CSF of patients with inflammatory brain diseases.

IL-6, originally described as a T-cell derived B-cell differentiation factor (B-cell stimulatory factor 2 = BSF-2),[11,12] plays an essential role in the terminal differentiation of B cells into antibody-secreting cells,[13] and stimulates the production of IgM, IgG, and IgA.[14-16]

MATERIALS AND METHODS

Patients

Paired CSF and serum specimens were collected by atraumatic lumbar puncture from 126 patients with various neurologic diseases. Forty patients had MS and were classified according to Poser *et al.*[17] The 12 patients having chronic (tension) headache showed normal physical and neurological examinations, and all paraclinical tests as well as routine blood and CSF analysis gave negative results.

The diagnosis of herpes-simplex virus type 1 (HSV-1) encephalitis, Lime's disease, neurosyphilis, and tubercolous meningitis were achieved by means of serological tests and/or by the isolation of the specific agent. Among the group of eight patients with degenerative diseases, two had Alzheimer's disease, two syringomyelia and four amyotrophic lateral sclerosis.

Patients with bacterial meningitis were not included in the study since we noticed that, at least in some CSF samples, bacterial products (eg, lipopolysaccaride) stimulated the proliferation of the 7TD1 cells; an activation of the B hybridoma cells not being neutralizable by anti-IL-6 antibodies.

Routine CSF Studies

The routine analysis of the CSF and the corresponding serum was performed as previously described in detail.[18,19] Briefly, after cell count and centrifugation, the concentration of albumin and IgG were measured by immunoprecipitation nephelometry. The blood-brain barrier (BBB) integrity was evaluated by calculating the CSF/serum albumin ratio,[20] while the quantitation of the intrathecal IgG synthesis was done by calculating the IgG index[20] and the intra-BBB IgG synthesis rate.[21] The demonstration of oligoclonal IgG bands in native or diluted CSF was carried out by means of agarose isoelectric focusing followed by nitrocellulose transfer of proteins, double immunofixation, avidin-biotin amplification, and peroxidase staining.

BSF-2/IL-6 Assay

The assay for BSF-2/IL-6 was performed using the BSF-2-dependent B-cell hybridoma 7TD1 (mouse-mouse) as previously described.[22] Briefly, 7TD1 cells (kindly provided by Dr J. van Snick, Ludwig Institute for Cancer Research, Brussels, Belgium) were seeded in 96-well microtiter F-plates in Iscove's modified Dulbecco's medium supplemented with 10% FCS, 5 x 10^{-5} M 2-ME, 1.5 mM L-glutamine, 0.24 mM L-asparigine, 0.55 mM L-arginine, and antibiotics.[23] The cells were cultured at a density of 10^3 cells per well in the presence of serial dilution of CSF or a highly purified standard containing 1000 U/ml of human BSF-2 (kindly provided by Dr J. van Damme, Rega Institute for Medical Research, University of Leuven, Belgium). For the final 16 hr or the 3-day culture, the cells were pulsed with 1 μCi [^{3}H]-thymidine (5 Ci/mmol). One unit of BSF-2 is defined as the amount of BSF-2 that results in half-maximal thymidine incorporation of the cells. When using highly purified BSF-2, the detection limit of BSF-2 was found to be 0.15 U/ml. When testing CSF, the detection limit of the BSF-2 assay was 10 U/ml due to negative effects of the samples when being tested at concentrations > 10%. To characterize the BSF-2-like activity in CSF, a neutralizing goat anti-human BSF-2 antibody was used[24] (a generous gift of Dr J. van Damme). After a 3 hr incubation of the samples with the antibody (final dilution 1:2000) at 37°C, the residual activity was determined in the assay.

RESULTS

BSF-2/IL-6 Activity in CSF

BSF-2 was found in 12 out of 15 CSF samples taken from patients with viral meningitis, and in all the CSF from patients with HSV-1 encephalitis and tubercolous meningitis (Fig. 1). Only rarely was this cytokine found in the CSF of patients with MS (2/40), subacute sclerosing panencephalitis (SSPE) (2/6), and Guillain-Barrè syndrome (2/12), while it was never detected in degenerative diseases of the CNS (0/8) nor in the CSF of patients with lumbar disk syndrome (0/14). All the positive CSF were completely neutralized by preincubation with a goat anti-human BSF-2 antiserum, demonstrating that the activity found was indeed due to CSF-2/IL-6 (Table 1).

Kinetics of BSF-2/IL-6 Production in Viral Meningitis

In some patients with viral meningitis it was possible to evaluate the correlation between the BSF-2 titers and the disease stage. These patients were chosen since they were not treated with anti-inflammatory or immunosuppressive drugs. The analysis of BSF-2 as a function of time showed a very early and tranient peak of the activity at the beginning of the disease, followed by an increase of the IgG indexes (Fig. 2).

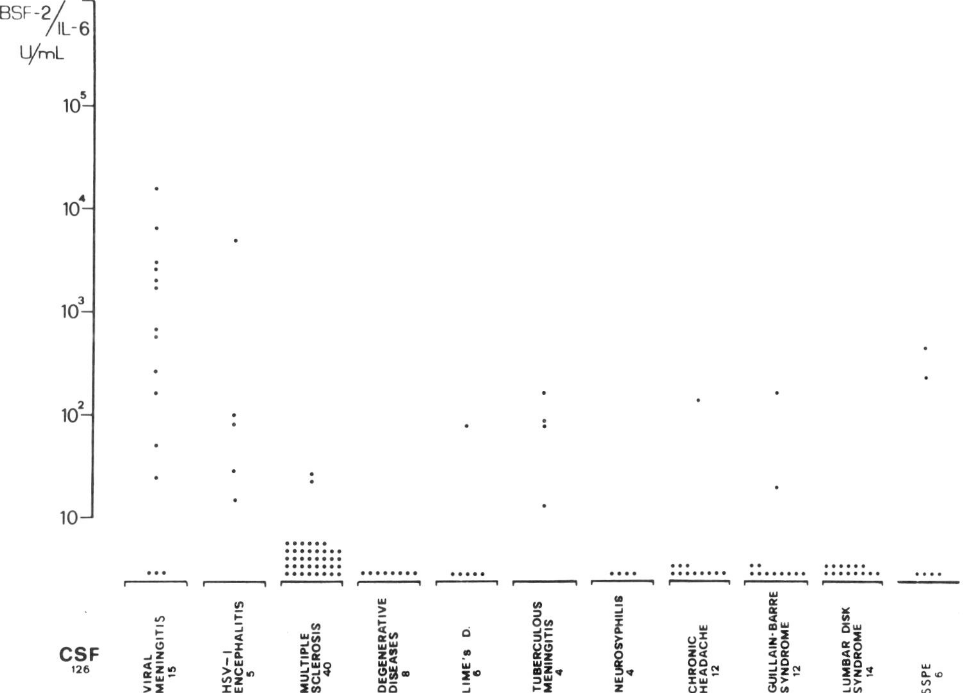

Fig. 1. BSF-2/IL-6 levels in the CSF of various neurologic diseases.

Correlation of BSF-2/IL-6 with other CSF Parameters

No correlation was found between BSF-2 titers and pleocytosis as well as between BSF-2 and the CSF/serum albumin ratio (index of BBB damage). Moreover, the BSF-2 levels did not correlate with the values of the IgG indexes (data not shown).

DISCUSSION

In the present study, considerable levels of BSF-2/IL-6 were found during the early stages of acute infections of the CNS (ie, viral meningitis, HSV-1 encephalitis). Moreover, this cytokine was demonstrated in all four CSF from patients with tubercolous meningitis (a chronic inflammation of the meninges). By contrast, this cytokine was only rarely demonstrated during the course of subacute and chronic inflammatory diseases of the central (MS, SSPE) and peripheral (Guillain-Barré syndrome) nervous system, and it was never detected in the CSF of patients with degenerative diseases.

The failure to detect this cytokine in the CSF of MS patients does not exclude its intracerebral production followed by complete assimilation at the target tissue level.

These findings are in agreement with an independent study previously reported.[25]

Recently we have detected BSF-2 also in CSF of mice infected intracerebrally with lymphocytic choriomeningitis virus.[22] The concentration of BSF-2 was

Table 1. Anti BSF-2 Antibodies Neutralize the BSF-2-like Activity Detected in CSF of Patients with Viral Meningitis, Tuberculous Meningitis and Multiple Sclerosis

Patients	(age/sex)	Disease	Dilution of CSF	Anti-BSF-2 Ab (1:2000)	Growth of 7TD1 cpm ± SD	Neutralization %
1	(3/F)	Viral meningitis	1 : 20	-	48,792 ± 785	86.5
				+	6,573 ± 336	
2	(24/F)	Tubercolous meningitis	1 : 10	-	37,792 ± 913	80.6
				+	7,346 ± 730	
3	(33/F)	Multiple sclerosis	1 : 20	-	14,642 ± 811	72.9
					3,385 ± 428	
BSF-2 standard			25 U/ml	-	52,908 ± 610	90.9
				+	4,813 ± 670	
7TD1 cells alone			-		5,799 ± 818	

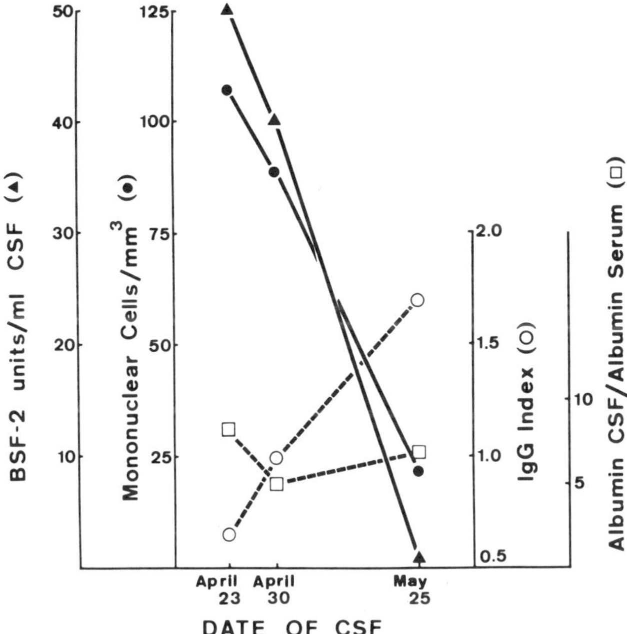

Fig. 2. Time-course of BSF-2/IL-6 in the CSF of a patient with viral meningitis, and its correlation with other CSF parameters.

about 60-fold higher in CSF compared with serum. These data suggest that BSF-2 is produced intrathecally.[22]

The presence of BSF-2/IL-6 in the CSF of acute viral infections may account for the intrathecal synthesis of antiviral antibodies that is commonly observed in these diseases in the form of increased IgG indexes and antiviral oligoclonal IgG. However, BSF-2 detected in CSF may also have other effects in the CNS. Recently it was found that BSF-2 cooperates with other soluble mediators in the differentiation of cytotoxic T lymphocytes[26] and granulocyte-macrophage progenitor cells.[27] Moreover, it acts on fibroblasts,[28] hepatocytes,[29] and thymocytes,[30] and induces fever when injected into experimental animals.[31]

Taken together, our data stress the possibility that many cell types, other than monocytes, may be capable of IL-6 production within the CNS.

ACKNOWLEDGEMENTS

This work was supported by grants from the Swiss National Science Foundation, the Swiss Multiple Sclerosis Society, and the European Science Foundation (P.G., 1988).

REFERENCES

1. M. A. Laurenzi and H. Link, Comparison between agarose gel electrophoresis and isoelectric focusing of CSF for demonstration of oligoclonal immunoglobulin bands in neurological disorders, *Acta Neurol.Scand.*, 58:148 (1978).

2. J. E. Olsson and K. Nelsson, Gamma globulins of CSF and serum in multiple sclerosis: isoelectric focusing of polyacrylamide gel and agar gel electrophoresis, *Neurology*, 29:1383 (1979).
3. E. J. Thompson, P. Kaufmann, and R. C. Shortan et al., Oligoclonal immunoglobulins and plasma cells in spinal fluid of patients with multiple sclerosis, *Brit.Med.J.*, 1:616 (1979).
4. H. Link, M. A. Laurenzi, and A. Fryden, Viral antibodies in oligoclonal and polyclonal IgG synthesized within the central nervous system over the course of mumps meningitis, *J.Neuroimmunol.*, 1:287 (1981).
5. D. H. Mattson, R. P. Roos, and B. G. W. Arnason, Comparison of agar gel electrophoresis and isoelectric focusing in multiple sclerosis and subacute sclerosing panencephalitis, *Ann.Neurol.*, 9:34 (1981).
6. V. Kostulas and H. Link, Agarose isoelectric focusing of unconcentrated CSF and radioimmunofixation for detection of oligoclonal bands in patients with multiple sclerosis and other neurological diseases, *J.Neurol.Sci.*, 454:17 (1982).
7. F. Vartdal, B. Vandvik, and T. E. Michaelsen, et al., Neurosyphilis: intrathecal synthesis of oligoclonal antibodies to treponema pallidum, *Ann.Neurol.*, 11:35 (1982).
8. F. Vartdal, B. Vandvik, and E. Norrby, Intrathecal synthesis of virus-specific oligoclonal IgG, IgA and IgM antibodies in a case of varicella-zoster meningoencephalitis, *J.Neurol.Sci.*, 57:121 (1982).
9. A. Henriksson, H. Link, M. Cruz, and G. Stiernstedt, Immunoglobulin abnormalities in cerebrospinal fluid and blood over the course of lymphocytic meningoradiculitis (Bannwarth's syndrome), *Ann.Neurol.*, 20:337 (1986).
10. E. Moller, H. Strom, and S. Al-Balaghi, Role of polyclonal activation in specific immune response. Relevance for findings of antibody activity in various diseases, *Scand.J.Immunol.*, 12:177 (1980).
11. T. Hirano, T. Taga, and N. Nakano, et al., Purification to homogeneity and characterization of human B-cell differentiation factor (BCDF or BSF-2), *Proc.Natl.Acad.Sci.* USA, 82: 5490 (1985).
12. M. Okada, N. Sakaguchi, and N. Toshimura, et al., B-cell growth factor (BCGF) and B-cell differentiation factor from human T hybridomas: two distinct kinds of BCGFs and synergism in B-cell proliferation, *J.Exp.Med.*, 157:583 (1983).
13. A. Muraguchi, T. Hirano, and B. Tang, et al., The essential role of B cell stimulatory factor 2 (BSF-2/IL-6) for the terminal differentiation of B cells, *J.Exp.Med.*, 167:332 (1988).
14. T. Hirano, K. Yasukawa, and H. Harada, et al., Complementary DNA for a novel human interleukin (BSF-2) that induces B lymphocytes to produce immunoglobulins, *Nature*, 324:73 (1986).
15. T. Kishimoto, Factors affecting B-cell growth and differentiation, *Ann.Rev.Immunol.*, 3:133 (1985).
16. P. B. Sehgal, L. T. May, I. Tamm, and J. Vilcek, Human β_2 interferon and B-cell differentiation factor BSF-2 are identical, *Science*, 124:731 (1987).
17. C. M. Poser, D. W. Paty, and L. Scheiderg, et al., New diagnostic criteria for multiple sclerosis: guidelines for research protocols, *Ann.Neurol.*, 13:227 (1983).
18. P. Gallo, F. Bracco, and B. Tavolato, Blood-brain-barrier damage restricts the reliability of quantitative formulae and isoelectric focusing in detecting intrathecally synthesized IgG, *J.Neurol.Sci.*, 84:87 (1988).
19. P. Gallo, F. Bracco, L. Battistin, and B. Tavolato, Detection of IgG oligoclonal bands in unconcentrated CSF by means of agarose isoelectric focusing, double immunofixation, peroxidase staining, and avidin-biotin amplification, *Ital.J.Neurol.Sci.*, 6:275 (1985).
20. G. Tibbling, H. Link, and S. Ohman, Principles of albumin and IgG analysis in neurological disorders. I. Establishment of reference values, *Scand.J.Clin.Lab.Invest.*, 37:385 (1977).

21. W. W. Tourtellotte, A. R. Potvin, and J. O. Fleming, et al., Multiple sclerosis: measurement and validation of central nervous system IgG synthesis rate, *Neurology*, 30:240 (1980).
22. K. Frei, T. P. Leist, and A. Meager, et al., Production of B-cell stimulatory factor-2 and interferon gamma in the central nervous system during viral meningitis and encephalitis, *J.Exp.Med.*, 168:449 (1988).
23. J. Van Snick, S. Cayphas, and A. Vink, et al., Purification and NH_2-terminal amino acid sequence of a T-cell derived lymphokine with growth factor activity for B-cell hybridoma, *Proc.Natl.Acad.Sci.* USA, 83:9679 (1986).
24. J. Van Damme, M. De Ley, and J. Van Snick, et al., The role of interferon β_1 and the 26 KDa protein (interferon $\beta 2$) as mediators of the antiviral effect of interleukin-1 and tumor necrosis factor, *J.Immunol.*, 139:1867 (1987).
25. F. A. Houssian, K. Bukasa, and C. J. M. Sindic, et al., Elevated levels of the 26K human hybridoma growth factor (interleukin-6) in cerebrospinal fluid of patients with acute infection of the central nervous system, *Clin.Exp.Immunol.*, 71:320-323 (1988).
26. Y. Yakai, G. G. Wong, and S. C. Clark, et al., B cell stimulatory factor 2 is involved in the differentiation of cytotoxic T lymphocytes, *J.Immunol.*, 140:508 (1988).
27. G. G. Wog, J. S. Witek-Gianotti, and P. A. Temple, et al., Stimulation of murine haemopoietic colony formation by human IL-6, *J.Immunol.*, 140:3040 (1988).
28. M. D. Kohase, D. Henriksen-Distefano, and L. T. May, et al., Induction of beta-2 interferon by tumor necrosis factor: a homeostatic mechanism in the control of cell proliferation, *Cell*, 45:659 (1986).
29. J. Gauldie, C. Richerds, and D. Harnish, et al., Interferon B-cell stimulatory factor type 2 shares identity with monocyte-derived hepatocyte-stimulating factor and regulates the major acute phase protein response in liver cells, *Proc.Natl.Acad.Sci.*, USE, 84:7251 (1987).
30. M. Lotz, F. Jirik, and P. Kabouridis, et al., B-cell stimulating factor 2/interleukin 6 is a costimulant for human thymocytes and T lymphocytes, *J.Exp.Med.*, 167:1253 (1988).
31. M. Helle, J. P. J. Brakenhoff, E. R. De Groot, and L. A. Aarden, Interleukin 6 is involved in interleukin 1-induced activities, *Eur.J.Immunol.*, 18:957-959 (1988).

Cell Studies

B-CELL RESPONSE EVALUATED AT CELLULAR LEVEL IN CSF AND BLOOD IN MULTIPLE SCLEROSIS AND CONTROLS

H. Link, S. Baig, Y.-P. Jiang, O. Olsson, B. Höjeberg, V. Kostulas and T. Olsson

Department of Neurology, Karolinska Institutet, Huddinge University Hospital, S-141 86 Huddinge, Stockholm, Sweden

ABSTRACT

When the B-cell response was examined by enumeration of immunoglobulin (Ig) secreting cells, normal cerebrospinal fluid (CSF) contained IgG secreting cells, indeed at an eight-fold higher proportion per 10^4 mononuclear cells (MNC) than blood. As expected, the proportion of IgG producing cells is mostly greatly increased in CSF from patients with multiple sclerosis (MS). Evaluation of antibody responses at cellular level (thereby bypassing probable drawbacks inherent in determinations of circulating antibody levels such as antibody binding to target) revealed that in one MS patient group, 57% had in CSF cells secreting IgG antibodies against myelin basic protein (MBP), and in another MS group, 55% had in CSF cells producing IgG antibodies against myelin-associated glycoprotein (MAG); both MBP and MAG are possible targets for immune attack in MS. Anti-MBP and anti-MAG IgG antibody secreting cells could occur in parallel or independently. They were rarely detected in blood, reflecting strong compartmentalization to CSF-CNS. Their possible role in MS pathogenesis is envisaged in light of recently suggested coupling between polyclonal B-cell hyperresponsiveness and antigen-driven specific response in autoimmune-prone individuals.

INTRODUCTION

Abnormalities related to B-cell axis are regularly demonstrable in CSF from patients with MS. These changes may reflect one of the major pathologic features of the disease, namely the inflammation which is predominated by perivascular accumulation of mononuclear cells (MNC). B-cell related CSF changes include intrathecal production of IgG with accentuated predominance of subclass gamma-1 and kappa light chains. This local IgG synthesis can be documented by elevated IgG index in about 75% and presence mostly in CSF exclusively of two or more oligoclonal bands in practically all patients with MS when CSF and simultaneously obtained serum are separated by electrophoresis or isoelectric focusing. These as well as other abnormalities, their establishment in a historical perspective and clinical applications have been the subject for recent extensive reviews.[1-3] Another important recent contribution in this context is the evaluation of quantitative determinations of free light chains in CSF in MS and controls.[4]

Here we present evidence that intrathecal immunoglobulin (Ig) synthesis is probably a normal phenomenon which is markedly escalated in MS; give results from evaluation of Ig and antibody production at single cell level; and discuss possible mechanisms for pathogenesis of MS in relation to multitude of antibodies produced intrathecally in MS.

IMMUNOGLOBULIN PRODUCTION IN NORMAL CSF

Synthesis of Ig within the CSF-CNS compartment has been considered to reflect a pathologic state in the form of an inflammatory reaction. This assumption implies that IgG level found in CSF under normal conditions reflects transudation of IgG from serum while elevated CSF IgG concentration is a result of either damage to the blood-brain barrier (BBB) or intra-BBB IgG synthesis, or both. However, intra-BBB synthesis of Ig as well as antibodies may be affected by a number of still less well defined factors such as (1) transudation from peripheral blood to CSF and clearance from CSF and peripheral blood, both of which might be influenced not only by the functional state of the BBB but also by the stereometric configuration and lipophilic properties of Ig etc; (2) metabolic rate or turnover which might be altered in different diseases; (3) binding of Ig to Fc receptors, of autoantibodies to target structures or of antibodies to exogenous or sequestrated and persisting microorganisms.

We have utilized a nitrocellulose immunospot assay to enumerate numbers of cells secreting Ig of different isotypes among MNC isolated from CSF (CSF-L) and peripheral blood (PBL). This immunospot assay[5,6] makes use of microtitre plates with wells of nitrocellulose bottoms.[7] For enumeration of IgG, IgA and IgM producing cells, wells are coated with heavy chain specific anti-human IgG, IgA or IgM. Aliquots containing 4-16 x 10^3 CSF-L or 10^5 PBL are applied into individual wells, and after incubation overnight, IgG, IgA or IgM secreting cells are visualized by immunostaining and counted.[2,8]

As 'normal' individuals, we have examined subjects with muscular tension headache, knowing that MNC are a normal constituent of CSF and occur at a mean value of 1.45 x 10^6/L, with a range of 0.3-6.2 among 38 subjects examined.[9] Contrary to previous belief, we found that CSF from 14 of 16 'normal' individuals (87%) contained IgG secreting cells at a mean value of 23 per 10^4 CSF-L (Table 1). Corresponding peripheral blood contained 1-6 (mean 3) IgG secreting cells per 10^4 MNC, which means that proportion of IgG secreting cells was about eight-fold higher in CSF than blood. IgA and IgM producing cells were also found in 'normal' CSF, but less frequently and at proportions similar to those found in blood.[10]

Inactive B-cells are restricted in their passage from peripheral blood to CSF, and occur at lower frequencies among MNC in CSF.[11-13] Our finding of 'activated' Ig secreting cells at higher frequency among CSF-L than PBL could be due to normal transfer of 'activated', subsequently IgG secreting B-cells through the BBB, or presence in normal CSF of factors which promote B-cell activation, differentiation and IgG secretion. The latter may be either a 'normal' phenomenon or triggered in the CSF-CNS compartment by normally occurring subclinically persisting viruses or other microorganisms.

IMMUNOGLOBULIN SECRETING CELLS IN CSF AND PERIPHERAL BLOOD IN MS

Assuming that numbers of cells secreting Ig should mirror the B-cell response in a more accurate way than concentrations of circulating Ig, we adopted a modified hemolytic protein A plaque assay to enumerate IgG, IgA and IgM secreting cells in CSF and peripheral blood. In one group of 37 MS patients, we found that cells secreting IgG, IgA and IgM were present in CSF at

Table 1. Numbers and Percentages of IgG, IgA and IgM Secreting Cells per 10^4 Mononuclear Cells Isolated from CSF and Peripheral Blood from 20 Subjects with Muscular Tension Headache.

		IgG		IgA		IgM	
		CSF	Blood	CSF	Blood	CSF	Blood
Absolute	Range	0-50	1-6	0-6	0-11	3-10	0-5
	Mean	23	3	2	3		1
	Median	19	4		2		
No. pos/ No. exam		14/16	20/20	7/13	19/20	2/9	9/20

frequencies of 89%, 70% and 57%, respectively. Quantitatively, there was a pronounced predominance per 10^4 CSF-L for IgG secreting cells. Elevated numbers of Ig producing cells were often found when corresponding CSF Ig levels, expressed as Ig index, were normal, indicating that enumeration of Ig producing cells in CSF has high sensitivity for documentation of an intrathecal B-cell response. We could also demonstrate that, as expected, IgG producing cells predominated in number in CSF in a majority of MS patients but, surprisingly, IgM or IgA producing cells predominated in 10 of 37 patients.[14-16]

NUMBERS OF ANTI-MBP ANTIBODY PRODUCING CELLS IN CSF AND BLOOD IN MS

Since myelin basic protein (MBP) can be used for induction of EAE and may appear in the CSF of patients with MS, and represents a possible target for immune attack in MS, much effort has been focused on demonstration in MS of antibodies directed against MBP. Based on use of a variety of methods, frequencies from 0-100% have been reported in MS CSF and serum.[17-23] To circumvent drawbacks related to determination of circulating anti-MBP antibodies, we adopted the nitrocellulose immunospot assay presented above, but used MBP for initial coating of the wells.[2,8]

When applying this assay to CSF-L and PBL from a group of 19 patients with MS, we found that 11 (57%) had in CSF cells secreting IgG antibodies against MBP (mean 14 per 10^4 CSF-L), constituting about 18% of IgG secreting cells in CSF.[24] Cells secreting MBP antibodies of IgA or IgM isotypes were demonstrable in 0 of 9 and 1 of 10 examined MS patients. This B-cell response was highly compartmentalized to CSF since no anti-MBP antibody secreting cells were demonstrable in peripheral blood even though the conditions for detection were better since at least 10^5 PBL were applied per well in contrast to 4 x 10^3 CSF-L. These data confirm that IgG antibodies against MBP may be produced in MS by CSF-L. Utilizing the same assay, we have preliminary data indicating that other chronic inflammatory nervous system disorders such as Lyme disease with neurological complications are frequently accompanied by presence of anti-MBP antibody secreting cells in CSF, while this is rarely seen in uncomplicated aseptic meningitis and has not been observed in muscular tension headache.

Hitherto, we have also examined nine patients with MS at two occasions 0.5-1 year apart for anti-MBP IgG antibody secreting cells in CSF and blood (Table 2). We have found pronounced fluctuations of numbers of these cells in CSF over the time course studied in some of the MS patients examined. Extended studies are warranted to allow conclusions regarding correlation to clinical and other laboratory variables, including magnetic resonance imaging data. In accordance with our initial findings, there was almost constant absence

Table 2. Numbers of Cells Secreting IgG Antibodies against MBP and Total Numbers of IgG Secreting Cells per 10^4 Mononuclear Cells of CSF and Peripheral Blood (PB) from Nine Untreated MS Patients Examined on Two Occasions 1/2-1 year Apart. Numbers within brackets denote anti-MBP IgG producing cells in % of total number of IgG secreting cells.

Patient No.	Mononuclear cells in CSF	IgG index (0.7)*	MBP-IgG CSF	MBP-IgG PB	Total IgG CSF	Total IgG PB
1:1	6	1.3	10 (35)	0	28	2
2	4	1.2	39 (35)	0.2	110	2
2:1	8	1.3	0 (0)	0	65	5
2	66	1.2	16 (4)	0	392	5
3:1	3	0.9	15 (100)	0	15	3
2	3	0.9	80 (80)	0	100	1
4:1	7	1.5	74 (28)	0	260	2
2	7	1.4	14 (29)	0	47	4
5:1	45	1.6	65 (36)	0	178	9
2	23	1.4	4 (5)	0	76	4
6:1	8	0.7	36	0	14	1
2	3	0.6	32	0	28	1
7:1	1	1.0	0	0	nd	5
2	1	1.4	0	0	20	3
8:1	9	1.5	0	0	77	3
2	9	1.4	7 (8)	0	85	2
9:1	6	1.1	26 (96)	0	27	1
2	9	1.3	32 (10)	0.3	310	6

* Upper reference limit.

of anti-MBP IgG producing cells in the patients' blood, and numbers of IgG producing cells in blood were similar to those registered in healthy subjects. These data confirm (1) the frequent occurrence of anti-MBP IgG antibody secreting cells in CSF, and (2) sequestration of the MBP IgG antibody response to CSF-CNS.

ENUMERATION OF CELLS IN CSF AND BLOOD SECRETING ANTIBODIES AGAINST MAG IN MS

Another potential target for immune attack in MS is myelin-associated glycoprotein (MAG). Anti-MAG antibodies have been reported in CSF from 70% of patients with MS,[20] while we have been unable to detect such antibodies in MS CSF when using sensitive ELISA. We have examined a group of 18 MS patients for the presence of cells secreting anti-MAG IgG antibodies, and found such cells in 10 patients (55%), with values varying between 0-62 (mean 7) per 10^4 CSF-L and constituting about 4% of IgG producing cells in CSF (Table 3). Three of the patients had low numbers of anti-MAG IgM antibodies in CSF. In peripheral blood, two patients (11%) had cells secreting anti-MAG IgG antibodies, and one IgM antibodies. All these 18 patients were again negative for anti-MAG IgG, IgA and IgM antibodies when examined by ELISA.

Table 3. Numbers of Cells Secreting IgG and IgM Antibodies against MAG, and Total Numbers of IgG and IgM Producing Cells per 10^4 Mononuclear Cells Isolated from CSF and Peripheral Blood (PB) from 18 Patients with Untreated MS

	MAG				Total			
	IgG		IgM		IgG		IgM	
	CSF	PB	CSF	PB	CSF	PB	CSF	PB
Range	0-62	0-0.3	0-8	0-0.8	18-522	2-6	0-7	0.1-18
Mean	7				153	5	2	2
No. pos/ No. exam	10/18	2/18	3/8	1/15	18/18	18/18	7/8	18/18

In analogy with the situation for anti-MBP antibodies, these studies confirm that a B-cell response directed against MAG may occur in MS and is to a major part compartmentalized to CSF-CNS. Among 30 control patients with a variety of other neurological diseases — but with exclusion of polyneuropathy — positive results for anti-MAG antibody secreting cells in CSF were rarely encountered, but control patient material needs to be expanded with larger groups with organic CNS diseases.

DO CELLS SECRETING IgG ANTIBODIES AGAINST MBP AND MAG OCCUR SIMULTANEOUSLY IN MS CSF?

In a few patients with MS, we have determined in parallel numbers of cells secreting IgG antibodies against MBP and MAG (Table 4). Five of the patients had, or lacked, in CSF both cell types, while in the remaining four either MBP or MAG IgG antibody secreting cells were demonstrable. This can be taken as one argument against a possibility that the MAG preparation which we used was contaminated with MBP. The compartmentalization of the immune response against MBP and MAG to CSF-CNS is obvious also for these nine patients.

ANTIBODY SPECIFICITIES RELATED TO FUNCTION

The diversity of antibody specificities demonstrated within the CSF-CNS in MS compared to the low diversity found in infectious nervous system diseases of known etiology such as SSPE, herpes simplex encephalitis or mumps meningitis, has resulted in the hypothesis that the B-cell hyperresponsiveness might represent 'nonsense' polyclonal B-cell activation (for a review see reference 25).

Table 4. Numbers of Cells Secreting IgG Antibodies against MAG and MBP, and of IgG Producing Cells per 10^4 Mononuclear Cells Isolated from CSF and Peripheral Blood (PB) from Nine Patients with Untreated MS. Numbers within brackets denote antibody producing cells in % of IgG producing cells

	MAG-IgG		MBP-IgG		Total IgG	
	CSF	PB	CSF	PB	CSF	PB
Range	0-62	0	0-42	0	34-522	2-6
Mean	13 (8)		15 (18)		124	4
No. pos/No. exam	5/9	0/9	7/9	0/9	9/9	9/9

On the other hand, most specific antibody responses start as polyclonal responses and are often accompanied by a large antigen-unrelated polyclonal component.[26] It has in fact not been possible to relate all, or in some instances even a major proportion of, oligoclonal IgG bands demonstrable in patients with nervous system infections such as mumps meningitis to mumps IgG antibodies[27] or neurological disorders associated with HIV infection to HIV IgG antibodies,[28] or to absorb all or even a majority of oligoclonal bands present in CSF and frequently also in serum from patients with HTLV-1 related myeloneuropathy by using HTLV-1 antigen preparations.[29] Polyclonal and specific antibody responses need not be mutually exclusive. Dziarsky[30] has proposed a model unifying initial polyclonal activation with subsequent antigen-driven specific response. The sequence of events could then be that, in autoimmune-prone individuals, B cells are intrinsically hyperresponsive to polyclonal activators and accessory signals, such as lymphokines. These B cells undergo initial activation, expansion, which also involves autoreactive clones, and differentiation into polyclonal antibody secreting cells — including autoantibodies — under the influence of exogenous or endogenous polyclonal activators. Infections, stress, trauma and other factors suspected to precipitate exacerbations of MS could be acting by these means, preferentially within the CSF-CNS compartment. Finally, because of the presence of autoantigens and lymphokines, produced by autoimmune-prone individuals either spontaneously or after polyclonal activation, the antigens and lymphokines cause further expansion of autoreactive B-cell clones, leading to dysfunction or destruction of target structures.

ACKNOWLEDGEMENTS

This work was partly supported by grants from the Swedish Medical Research Council (project No. 3381). We thank Ms Yvonne Nilsson for help in preparing this manuscript.

REFERENCES

1. W. W. Tourtellotte, The cerebrospinal fluid in multiple sclerosis, *in*: "Handbook of Clinical Neurology", vol 3:47 J.C. Koetsier, ed., pp 79-130, Elsevier, Amsterdam (1985).
2. H. Link, CSF IgG and its congeners, *in*: "Advances in CSF Protein Research and Diagnosis", E.J. Thompson, ed., pp 49-88, MTP Press, Lancaster (1987).
3. H. Link, Cerebrospinal fluid in immunological CNS diseases, *in*: "Clinical Neuroimmunology", J.A. Aarli, W.M.H. Behan and P.O. Behan, eds, pp 444-466, Blackwell, Oxford (1987).
4. O. C. Fagnart, C. J. M. Sindic, and C. Laterre, Free kappa and lambda light chain levels in the cerebrospinal fluid of patients with multiple sclerosis and other neurological diseases, *J.Neuroimmunol.*, 19:119-132 (1988).
5. C. C. Czerkinsky, L. A. Nilsson, and H. Nygren, A solid-phase enzyme-linked immunospot (ELISPOT) assay for enumeration of specific antibody-secreting cells, *J.Immunol.Meth.*, 65:109-121 (1983).
6. J. D. Sedgewick and P. G. Holt, A solid-phase immunoenzymatic technique for the enumeration of specific antibody secreting cells, *J.Immunol. Meth.*, 57:301-309 (1983).
7. S. A. Möller and C. A. R. Borrebaeck, A filter immunoplaque assay for the detection of antibody-secreting cells *in vitro*, *J.Immunol.Meth.*, 79:195-204 (1985).
8. H. Link, S. Baig, T. Olsson, and F. Lolli, Antibody producing cells in CSF: A new tool for evaluation of B cell response in MS, *in*: "Trends in European Multiple Sclerosis Research", C. Confavreux, G. Aimard and M. Devic, eds, pp 173-181, Excerpta Medica, Amsterdam (1988).
9. S. Sörnäs and H. Ostlund, The cytology of the cerebrospinal fluid, *Acta Neurol.Scand.*, 48:313 (1972).

10. H. Link, S. Baig, V. Kostulas, and T. Olsson, Immunoglobulin-secreting cells in cerebrospinal fluid from patients with muscular tension headache, *J.Neuroimmunol.*, in press.
11. J. Ernerudh, T. Olsson, G. Berlin, B. Gustafsson, and H. Karlsson, Cell surface markers for diagnosis of central nervous system involvement in lymphoproliferative diseases, *Ann.Neurol.*, 20:610-615 (1986).
12. J. Ernerudh, S. Fredriksson, T. Olsson, and P. Forsberg, Leukocyte types in cerebrospinal fluid and peripheral blood enumerated immunoenzymatically in aseptic meningitis and Guillain-Barré syndrome, *Acta Neurol.Scand.*, 79:68-74 (1989).
13. S. Fredrikson, J. Ernerudh, T. Olsson, P. Forsberg, and H. Link, Mononuclear cell types in multiple sclerosis CSF and blood quantitated by immunoenzyme with panel of monoclonal antibodies, *Arch.Neurol.*, 46:372-375 (1989).
14. A. Henriksson, S. Kam-Hansen, and R. Andersson, Immunoglobulin-producing cells in CSF and blood from patients with multiple sclerosis and other inflammatory neurological diseases enumerated by protein A plaque assay, *J.Neuroimmunol.*, 1:299-309 (1981).
15. A. Henriksson, S. Kam-Hansen, and H. Link, IgM, IgA and IgG producing cells in cerebrospinal fluid and peripheral blood in multiple sclerosis, *Clin.exp.Immunol.*, 62:176-184 (1985).
16. A. Henriksson, Immunoglobulin producing cells in nervous system diseases, *Acta Neurol.Scand.*, 73: suppl 104, 1-109 (1986).
17. H. S. Panitch, C. J. Hooper, and K. P. Johnson, CSF antibody to myelin basic protein. Measurement in Patients with multiple sclerosis and subacute sclerosing panencephalitis, *Arch.Neurol.*, 37:206-209 (1980).
18. B. Roström, Specificity of antibodies in oligoclonal bands in patients with multiple sclerosis and cerebrovascular disease, *Acta Neurol.Scand.*, 63: suppl 86, 1-84 (1981).
19. C.-H. Chou, W. W. Tourtellotte, and R. F. Kibler, Failure to detect antibodies to myelin basic protein in CSF of patients with MS, *Neurology*, 33:24-28 (1983).
20. A. Wajgt and M. Gorny, CSF antibodies to myelin basic protein and to myelin-associated glycoprotein in multiple sclerosis. Evidence of the intrathecal production of antibodies, *Acta Neurol.Scand.*, 68:337-343 (1983).
21. E. Alvord, S. Hruby, C. M. Shaw, and J. Slimp, Myelin basic protein and its antibodies in the cerebrospinal fluid in experimental allergic encephalomyelitis, multiple sclerosis and other diseases, *in*: "Experimental Allergic Encephalomyelitis: A Useful Model for Multiple Sclerosis", E. Alvord, M. Kies and A. Suckling, eds, pp 359-365, Alan R. Liss Inc. (1984).
22. M. Cruz, T. Olsson, J. Ernerudh, B. Höjeberg, and H. Link, Immunoblot detection of oligoclonal antimyelin basic protein IgG antibodies in cerebrospinal fluid in multiple sclerosis, *Neurology*, 37:1515-1519 (1987).
23. P. Matsiota, A. Blancher, B. Doyon, B. Guilbert, M. Clanet, E. D. Kouvelas, and S. Avrameas, Comparative study of natural autoantibodies in the serum and cerebrospinal fluid of normal individuals and patients with multiple sclerosis and other neurological diseases, *Ann.Inst.Pasteur/Immunol.*, 139:99-108 (1988).
24. T. Olsson, S. Baig, B. Höjeberg, and H. Link, Quantitation of anti-myelin basic protein and anti-myelin antibody producing cells in multiple sclerosis and controls, *Ann.Neurol.*, in press.
25. T. A. Reder and B. G. W. Arnason, Immunology of multiple sclerosis, *in*: "Handbook of Clinical Neurology, vol 3 (47): Demyelinating Diseases", J.C. Koetsier, ed., pp 337-395, Elsevier, Amsterdam (1985).
26. Y. Rosenberg and J. M. Chiller, Ability of antigen-specific helper cells to effect a class-restricted increase in total Ig-secreting cells in spleens after immunization with the antigen, *J.Exp.Med.*, 150:517-530 (1979).

27. H. Link, M. Laurenzi, and A. Frydén, Viral antibodies in oligoclonal and polyclonal IgG synthesized within the central nervous system over the course of mumps meningitis, *J.Neuroimmunol.*, 1:287-298 (1981).
28. K. S.-S. Bukasa, C. J. M. Sindic, M. Bodeus, C. Laterre, and J. Sonnet, Anti-HIV antibodies in the CSF of AIDS patients: a serological and immunoblotting study, *J.Neurol.Neurosurg.Psychiat.*, 51:1063-1068 (1988).
29. H. Link, M. Cruz, A. Gessain, O. Gout, G. de Thé, and S. Kam-Hansen, Chronic progressive myelopathy associated with HTLV-I IgG antibody patterns in cerebrospinal fluid and srum, *Neurology*, in press.
30. R. Dziarski, Autoimmunity: polyclonal activation or antigen induction? *Immunol.Today*, 11:340-342 (1988).

ANTIOLIGODENDROCYTE AUTOREACTIVE T CELLS

V. Jewtoukoff and M. A. Bach

Unité de Pathologie de l'Immunité, Institut Pasteur,
25 rue du Dr Roux, 75724 Paris Cedex 15, France

SUMMARY

We have investigated the role of oligodendrocytes (OD), the glial cells that produce the myelin sheath in the central nervous system (CNS), as possible targets for T-cell mediated autoimmune demyelinating processes.

In a first set of experiments, lymph node cells (LNC) from SJL/J mice immunized with either rat whole spinal cord (WSC) homogenate or myelin basic protein (BP) in the presence of complete Freund's adjuvant (CFA) were assayed for their *in vitro* proliferative response to BP and to purified OD. WSC-immunized mice displayed a strong and persistent response to both syngeneic and rat OD, and a much weaker response to rat BP. Moreover LNC from BP-immunized mice showed a small response to BP, but no response to OD, indicating that OD are not able to present their endogeneous BP to lymphocytes. These data suggest that autoreactive T cells, specific for OD antigens other than BP, had been stimulated by WSC-immunization.

To further characterize these T cells, a second set of experiments was undertaken, where normal SJL/J mouse splenocytes were sensitized *in vitro* by Lewis rat OD and maintained as long-term T cell lines in IL-2-containing medium. These lines were initially composed of a majority of CD4+ CD8- T cells and could mount a proliferative response to Lewis rat OD in the absence of IL-2. T cell lines cultured for more than 4 months included a majority of CD8+ CD4- T cells and required exogeneous IL-2 to develop a proliferative response to OD. A T cell clone of the CD8+ CD4- phenotype was obtained from these lines. The proliferative response of these lines and clones could be elicited by syngeneic OD as well as by Lewis rat OD, but appeared to be tissue-specific, since other tissues failed to trigger their proliferation, and was not MHC-restricted.

The molecular nature of the OD autoantigen recognized, and the pathogenic and/or physiologic role of these non-classical autoreactive T cells remain to be elucidated.

INTRODUCTION

Although myelin basic protein (BP) represents a major autoantigen in the model of experimental allergic encephalomyelitis (EAE),[1] other myelin components also play a role in autoimmune demyelinating diseases. Thus, EAE can be induced by proteolipid apoprotein (PLP), as well as by BP, either by active immunization or by passive transfer of antigen-specific activated CD4 T cells.[2,3] Autoantibodies to galactocerebroside C (Gal C) or to MOGOM2 myelin glycoprotein, both markers expressed at the surface of oligodendrocytes, were shown to act in synergy with BP-specific T cells in the process of demyelination.[4-7] The way these autoantigens can activate autoreactive T cells is not clear, since glial cells do not constitutively express class II antigens of the major histocompatibility complex (MHC),[8] which are normally required for antigen recognition by CD4 T cells.[9] Astrocytes, microglial cells and endothelial cells may however express MHC class II antigens upon stimulation by gamma interferon and may serve as antigen-presenting cells for preactivated T cells.[10] Resting oligodendrocytes do not express any MHC antigen, and seem to acquire only class I MHC antigen expression when stimulated by gamma interferon.[8] On the other hand, they do synthesize most of the autoantigens that have proven to be relevant to autoimmune demyelinating processes. It seemed therefore interesting to us to explore their possible role as target cells for antimyelin autoimmunity. The data presented in this study indicate that oligodendrocyte-specific autoreactive T cells represent a major component of the T cell response to whole spinal cord immunization and that some autoreactive T cells, isolated and cloned from normal mouse spleen, can recognize their OD target without MHC restriction.

MATERIALS AND METHODS

Animals

Lewis rats and SJL/J mice were obtained from the animal breeding unit of the Pasteur Institute (Paris, France).

Immunization

SJL/J mice aged 6-8 weeks were immunized into the hind footpads with either rat MBP (100 μg) (kindly given by Dr G. Hashim, St Luke's Roosevelt Hospital Center, NY, USA) or WSC (10 mg) in CFA. Each mouse also received two iv injections of 6 x 10^9 *Bordetella pertussis* (Pasteur Institute, Paris, France) on Day 0 and Day 2. Mice were killed on Day 30; their popliteal lymph nodes were removed and a single cell suspension was prepared, to assess the proliferative response of lymph node cells to BP and glial cells as described below.

Preparation of Cell Suspensions

OD and astrocyte suspensions were prepared according to the method of Hirayama et al,[11] and McCarthy et al,[12] respectively. Spleen and lymph node cells were prepared by gentle teasing, and kidney cells were obtained by kidney cortex dissection and trypsinization. Cells were resuspended in culture medium consisting of Dulbecco's minimum essential medium, containing 2 mM L-glutamine, 1 mM sodium pyruvate, 1 mM non-essential aminoacids, 5 x 10^{-5} M 2-mercaptoethanol and 100 UI/ml of penicillin-streptomycin, supplemented with 10% heat-inactivated fetal calf serum. Twenty μg/ml of bovine insulin and 5 mg/ml of glucose were added for glial cell cultures.

Establishment of OD-specific T Cell Lines and Clones

SJL/J mouse spleen cells (SC) suspended in culture medium were plated onto Lewis rat OD primary cultures. After a 10 to 12-day culture, Con A-stimulated rat SC supernatant was added as a source of interleukine 2 (IL-2). The T cell lines were then maintained for *in vitro* long-term culture with IL-2-supplemented medium and restimulating by Lewis rat OD once a month. These T cell lines were cloned by limiting dilution in Terasaki plates, containing irradiated (50 Gy) Lewis rat OD in a final volume of 10 μl IL-2-supplemented medium. A single growing colony, named C2, could be further subcloned and expanded as the T cell lines.

In Vitro Proliferation Assays

Long-term cultured T-cells (5×10^3) were incubated in triplicates with 5×10^4 irradiated (50 Gy) OD from various sources in 0.2 ml culture medium in 96-well round bottomed microtiter plates as described elsewhere.[13] As controls, the same T cells were tested without antigen, or with 5×10^4 irradiated (50 Gy) other stimulating cells such as syngeneic, allogeneic or xenogeneic SC, Con A- and LPS-activated lymphoblasts, kidney cells and astrocytes. Proliferative response to rat myelin BP (50 µg/ml) was also tested in presence of syngeneic irradiated (50 Gy) SC used as antigen-presenting cells. Cultures were pulsed by 0.037 MBq/well of methyl [^{3}H]-thymidine at 48 hr except when otherwise stated, and were harvested 18 hr later by using an automatic cell harvester. Beta radioactivity was measured in a liquid scintillation counter. A proliferative response was considered significant when the stimulation index (cpm with antigen/cpm without antigen) was ≥ 2, and when the mean cpm obtained with and without antigen were statistically different ($p < 0.05$) as assessed by '*t*' test.

Freshly isolated lymph node cells were tested for their proliferative responses following the same procedures, except that cultures were performed with 2×10^5 cells in flat-bottomed culture plates, and lasted for 5 days.

Phenotypic Analysis of T Cells

T cells were stained by indirect immunofluorescence as described elsewhere[13] with monoclonal antibodies (mAb) directed against anti-Lyt-2.2 (CD8), mAb anti-L_3T_4 (CD4) and mAb anti CD3. Second antibody consisted in FITC-goat anti-mouse Ig, prepared in our laboratory. Cells were examined either under the Leitz fluorescence microscope or by flow cytometry with a FACS Analyzer (Becton and Dickinson).

RESULTS AND DISCUSSION

WSC-Immunized SJL/J Mice Develop an Autoreactive Anti-OD Lymphocyte Response

As shown in Table 1, LNC from mice immunized with rat WSC (plus CFA) could mount a proliferative response to both mouse syngeneic OD and rat OD that was much higher than that elicited by rat BP. A smaller but significant response to rat splenocytes (but not to syngeneic splenocytes) suggested the existence of some T cell response to widely distributed rat xenoantigens beside the tissue-specific response to OD. Sonication of OD prior to testing nearly abrogated the cell proliferative response, which is therefore most likely directed against OD surface antigens (data not shown).

On the other hand, LNC from mice immunized with BP+CFA developed a proliferative response to BP only, and not to OD. Thus OD, in contrast to Schwann cells[14] are not able to present their endogeneous BP to BP-reactive T cells. Neither the nature of the OD antigen that elicit the lymphocyte proliferative response in WSC-immunized animals, nor the pathogenic role of the OD-triggered proliferation, are known. Among membrane-expressed OD antigens, the glycoprotein MOG/M2 is a possible candidate, since it elicits high level of IgG antibodies in animals in which EAE is actively induced by WSC immunization.[4,6]

The relative contribution of T and B cells to the proliferative response to OD was not precisely defined, but T cells most likely play a major role since: (1) depletion of B cells from WSC- and BP-sensitized LNC through nylon-wool columns did not reduce the proliferative response to OD of the remaining T cells

Table 1. Preferential Proliferative Response to Oligodendrocytes of Lymphocytes from Whole Spinal Cord-sensitized Mice

	Antigens					
Responding cells	None	B P	Lewis rat O D	SJL/J mouse O D	Lewis rat S C	SJL/J mouse S C
WSC-sensitized LNC	4228	10303* (2.44)	106116 (25.1)	108616 (25.6)	27585 (6.5)	3729 (0.9)
BP-sensitized LNC	3789	11154 (2.9)	4115 (1.1)	1915 (0.5)	4547 (1.2)	3083 (0.8)

* Mean of triplicates. [^{3}H]-thymidine incorporation was measured on Day 5 of culture after an 18 hour pulse. Values significantly different from those of unstimulated cultures are underlined. Stimulation indexes (= cpm of antigen stimulated cultures/cpm of unstimulated cultures) are shown in parentheses.

Table 2. Oligodendrocyte-specific Proliferative Response of OD-triggered T Cell Line and Clone

		Antigens					
Responding cells	IL-2	None	Lewis rat OD	SJL/J mouse OD	Lewis rat SC	SJL/J mouse SC	Lewis rat kidney cells
OD-triggered T cell line	-	297*	<u>4594</u>	<u>3011</u>	1191	105	nd
T cell clone C2	-	111	209	207	182	73	392
	+	3543	<u>17423</u>	<u>14775</u>	4538	6909	2717
Fresh SJL/J mouse SC	-	85	285	215	151	123	1021
	+	117	551	399	375	361	968

* Mean of triplicates. [^{3}H]-thymidine incorporation was measured on Day 3 of culture after an 18 hour pulse. Values significantly different from those of unstimulated cultures are underlined. nd = not done.

(data not shown); and (2) *in vitro* cellular proliferative responses to most antigens are correlated with *in vivo* cell-mediated immunity and generally require T cell activation.[15]

A contribution of B-cells is however not excluded since WSC-immunization was shown to trigger the production of large amounts of autoantibodies to OD[16] or to some OD surface components such as M2/MOG and Gal C.[4,17]

Normal SJL/J Mouse Harbour Anti-OD, Tissue-specific, Autoreactive T Cells which are not MHC Restricted

As we described elsewhere,[13] OD-specific T cell lines and one OD-specific T cell clone could be isolated from the spleen of normal, non-immunized SJL/J mice, by *in vitro* sensitization over Lewis rat OD monolayers and expansion in IL2-containing medium. Polyclonal T cell lines were first obtained. As shown in Table 2, these lines specifically proliferated in the presence of both syngeneic and rat OD, but not in the presence of other rat or mouse tissues. OD were neither able to stimulate a significant proliferative response of fresh, unselected T cells, and thus do not act as non-specific polyclonal activators.

As long as the T cell lines comprised a majority of CD4 T cells (that is during the first 4 months of culture), their proliferative response to OD did not require the addition of exogeneous IL2 to the medium, probably because these lines themselves produced IL2 in response to antigenic stimulation. Over time, OD-specific T cell lines get enriched in CD8+ T cells and became dependent on exogeneous IL2 to mount an OD-specific proliferative response.

At that time, a T cell clone was selected from OD-specific T cell lines by limiting dilution. As shown in Table 2, it also expressed an OD-specific, IL2-dependent, proliferative response to both syngeneic and rat OD, and was found to be a CD3+, CD8+, CD4- T cell. From these experiments, it appears that normal mice harbour tissue-specific, autoreactive T cells that can proliferate to OD in a non-species restricted manner. This lack of restriction by self MHC antigens was further confirmed by the observation that the T cell clone C2 could also proliferate to guinea-pig OD, as well as to OD from various allogeneic mouse strains.[13] Although the requirement for antigen-specific T cells to recognize epitopes in association with self MHC antigens is widely accepted as a rule,[9] several exceptions have been described. Indeed, Wakabayashi et al[18] reported tissue-specific mouse T cells that were cytolytic to both syngeneic melanomas and human melanomas; Boitard et al[19] identified in patients with type 1 diabetes, circulating CD8 T cells that could recognize rat Langherans islet β cells but not α cells.

Whether these 'natural' autoreactive T cells do contribute to the T cell proliferative response triggered by rat WSC-immunization against syngeneic OD remains unknown but is a likely possibility. Whether they play a physiologic role in non-immunized animals and/or a pathogenic role in WSC-immunized animals has to be explored.

REFERENCES

1. C. C. A. Bernard and P. R. Carnegie, *J.Immunol.*, 114:1537-1540 (1975).
2. P. K. Olitsky and C. Tal, *Proc.Soc.Exp.Biol.Med.*, 79:50-56 (1952).
3. J. Satoh, K. Sakai, M. Endoh, F. Koike, T. Kunishita, T. Namikawa, T. Yamamura, and T. Tabira, *J.Immunol.*, 138:179-184 (1987).
4. R. Lebar, C. Vincent, and E. Fisher-Le Boubennec, *J.Neurochem.*, 32:1451-1460 (1979).
5. C. Linington, M. Webb, and P. L. Woodham, *J.Neuroimmunol.*, 6:387-396 (1984).

6. R. Lebar, C. Lubetski, C. Vincent, P. Lombrail, and J. M. Boutry, *Clin.Exp. Immunol.*, 66:423-443 (1986).
7. H. J. Schluesener, R. A. Sobel, C. Linington, and H. L. Weiner, *J.Immunol.*, 139:4016-4021 (1987).
8. A. Suzumura, D. H. Silberberg, and R. P. Lisak, *J.Neuroimmunol.*, 11:179-190 (1986).
9. J. L. Strominger, *Prog.Immun.*, 4:541-554 (1980).
10. A. Fontana and W. Fierz, Springer, *Sem.Immunopathol.*, 8:17-70 (1985).
11. M. Hirauama, D. Silberberg, R. Lisak, and D. Pleasure, *J.Neuropath.Exp. Neurol.*, 42:16-28 (1983).
12. K. D. McCarthy and J. de Cellis, *J.Cell.Biol.*, 85:890-902 (1980).
13. V. Jewtoukoff and M. A. Bach, *J.Autoimmunity*, in press.
14. H. Wekerle, M. Schwab, C. Linington, and R. Meyermann, *Eur.J.Immunol.*, 16:1551-1557 (1986).
15. H. J. Meuwissen, P. J. Van Alten, and R. A. Good, 102:1079-1083 (1969).
16. O. Abramsky, *J.Med.Sci.*, 18:149-158 (1982).
17. C. S. Raine, A. B. Johnson, P. Marcus, A. Suzuki, and M. B. Bornstein, *J. Neurol.Sci.*, 52:117-131 (1981).
18. S. Wakabayashi, M. Taniguchi, T. Tokuhisa, H. Tomioka, and S. Okamoto, *Nature*, 294:748-750 (1981).
19. C. Boitard, L. Chatenoud, and M. Debray-Sachs, *J.Immunol.*, 129:2529-2531 (1982).

IMBALANCE OF CSF LYMPHOCYTE SUBSETS IN MULTIPLE SCLEROSIS

Maria Giovanna Marrosu

Instituto di Neuropsichiatria Infantile
Università, via Ospedale 119
I-09124 Cagliari, Italy

Immunological involvement in multiple sclerosis (MS) has been clearly established. In particular, the presence of T cells infiltrating MS brain parenchima has been reported,[1-3] suggesting a process of immune-mediated damage. However, two major questions are still unresolved: first, if the reported cellular infiltrates constitute the basis of the MS lesions and, second, if an *in vivo* study of T cell traffic occurring in the central nervous system (CNS) is possible. These two questions are strictly linked, since answering the second one may shed some light on interpreting MS pathogenetic mechanisms. In this respect, the study of cerebrospinal fluid (CSF) cells may represent a way to elucidate the role of lymphocyte infiltrates found in post-mortem MS brains.

There is considerable evidence that immune response in CNS occurs in partial isolation from the peripheral compartment. In fact, peripherally activated lymphocytes can cross the blood-brain barrier, whereas resting lymphocytes cannot;[4] if activated lymphocytes encounter the same antigen, they proliferate within the CNS. In addition, immune surveillance in the CNS takes place following its own rules driven by immune reactions induced in neural tissue by lymphokines secreted by activated lymphocytes. Therefore, we can suppose that CSF cells may reflect immune reaction within the CNS more exactly than peripheral blood (PB) cells. For this reason, we studied CSF lymphocyte subsets to elucidate the role of immune mediated cells in MS pathogenesis.

In our previous studies, using the rosette forming-cells method, we found a reduction in CSF EA-rosette (Tγ cells, ie, cells having suppressor or cytotoxic activity,[5] in MS: we hypothesized, therefore, a loss of suppressor activity in MS.

Using monoclonal antibody (mAb) technique, we were unable to find significant differences in CSF lymphocyte subsets from a small sample of MS patients compared to subjects with other neurological diseases,[6] while in a second report we found some variations in the percentages of CSF MS cells in relation to the state of the disease and to clinical symptomatology.[7]

The present report shows the results of our latest studies concerning the evaluation of T3, T4, T8 and T3/T8 ratio, DR and IL-2R positive CSF cells in MS. Moreover, we report experiments by the dual fluorescence method using anti-2H4 and anti-4B4 mAbs.

MATERIALS AND METHODS

Patients

We studied 47 definite (Rose's criteria,[8] MS patients (35 females and 12 males, mean age 30.5 years, range 12-38) without therapy for at least one month, 45 of them with a relapsing-remitting course (42 in acute relapse and three in stable phase) and two had a progressive form from onset.

Twenty-one subjects affected with various non immunological diseases (NID) and 14 with inflammatory diseases of the central nervous system (ID) were used as comparison.

CSF Cell Isolation

Immediately after sterile lombar puncture, 6-10 ml of CSF without blood contamination were centrifuged for 10 min at 1200 g in a glass sterile tube. The supernatant was gently removed and used for routine analysis. The cells contained in the pellet (1 ml) were counted by Nageotte chamber.

Monoclonal Antibodies (mAbs)

Five µl of anti-T3 (total T cells), anti-T4 (T helper/inducer), anti-T8 (T suppressor/cytotoxic), anti-DR (HLA-DR determinant), anti-NK (NK cells), all available from Ortho Diagnostic System (USA) and 2 µl of anti-IL-2R (anti-IL-2 receptor, T activated cells) by Becton-Dickinson (Erembodegen, Belgium) were used. Al mAbs were FITC conjugated. Moreover, anti-2H4 and anti-4B4 (Coulter Immunology, Hialeah, Flo.) phycoerylthrin conjugated mAbs were used for two-color fluorescence analysis: the former mAb reacted with approximately 42% of T4+ inducer cells and 54% of T8 cytotoxic/suppressor population,[9] and the latter with approximately 41% of T4+ inducer subset and 43% of T8 cytotoxic/suppressor population.[10]

Flow Cytometry

Single-color fluorescence analysis was used in performing flow cytometry with a Spectrum III cell sorter (Ortho Diagnostic System, USA). Two color fluorescence analysis was carried out on a Spectrum III cell sorter equipped with a dual laser (argon wavelength, 488 nm for fluorescin-isothiocyanate and krypton wavelength, 568 nm for Texas red). For each sample, at least 100 cells were examined on a logarithmic scale and elaborated by DS-1 (Ortho). All analyses were performed without knowledge of the clinical diagnosis.

Statistical Analysis

Student's *t* test was used.

RESULTS

(1) T3, T4, T8, NK CSF cell subsets and T4/T8 ratio in MS patients compared to NID (Table 1): significantly high percentages of T4+ ($p<0.05$) and low percentages of T8+ ($p<0.02$) cells (with consequent high T4/T8 ratio, $p<0.001$) were found in MS CSF samples.

(2) T3, T4, T8, NK CSF cell subsets and T4/T8 ratio in MS patients compared to ID (Table 1): significantly high percentages of T4+ cells, high T4/T8 ratio ($p<0.001$) and high percentages of NK cells ($p<0.05$) were found in MS CSF samples.

Table 1. Percentages of cerebrospinal fluid cell subsets in multiple sclerosis (MS), non immunological (NID) and inflammatory diseases (ID) of the central nervous system

	T3	T4	T8	T4/T8	NK
MS					
M	70.3	50.0	20.4	3.5	21.8
+SD	18.2	15.1	9.1	2.4	16.1
n	45	45	45	45	23
NID					
M	59.9	40.1	29.8	1.2	12.2
+SD	23.1	15.3	12.9	0.4	20.8
n	11	11	11	11	16
ID					
M	69.3	33.6	21.1	1.8	10.9
+SD	12.9	14.0	11.0	0.9	12.3
n	12	14	14	14	13

Significant differences (Student's *t* test)
MS vs NID: T4 $p<0.05$; T8 $p<0.02$; T4/T8 $p<0.001$
MS vs ID: T4 $p<0.001$; T4/T8 $p<0.001$; NK $p<0.05$

Table 2. Percentages of cerebrospinal fluid activated cells in multiple sclerosis (MS), non immunological (NID) and inflammatory diseases (ID) of the central nervous system

		DR	IL - 2R
MS	M ± SD	19.5 ° 16.0	2.0 ± 2.5*
	n	45	45
NID	M ± SD	14.8 ± 13.7	0.5 ° 1.6
	n	19	17
ID	M ± SD	15.3 ± 13.1	2.3 ± 3.7
	n	14	9

Significant differences (Student's t test): * $p<0.025$

Table 3. Percentages of cerebrospinal fluid T4+2H4+, T8+2H4+, T4+2H4+/T4 and T8+2H4+/T8+ subsets in multiple sclerosis (MS) and other neurological diseases (OND)

	T4+2H4+	T8+2H4+	T4+2H4+/T4	T8+2H4+/T8+
MS	27.2	12.4	58.2	64.4
+SD	14.3	9.5	23.6	36.2
n	22	10	22	10
			*	†
OND				
M	25.5	14.4	82.6	95.6
+SD	12.3	10.5	19.2	9.9
n	9	5	9	5

Significant differences (*t* test): * $p<0.001$; † $p<0.025$.

Table 4. Percentages of cerebrospinal fluid T4+4B4+, T8+4B4+, T4+4B4+/T4+ and T8+4B4+/T8+ subsets in multiple sclerosis (MS) and other neurological diseases (OND)

	T4+2B4+	T8+4B4+	T4+4B4+/T4	T8+4B4+/T8+
MS				
M	44.7	19.7	89.8	94.0
+SD	12.8	7.1	10.2	9.8
n	22	10	22	10
	†	*		
OND				
M	35.6	7.4	91.3	99.1
+SD	10.3	5.6	18.1	2.1
n	9	5	9	5

Significant differences (*t* test): * $p<0.005$; † $p<0.05$.

(3) DR+ and IL-2R+ cells in MS patients compared to NID and ID (Table 2): significantly high percentages of ($p<0.025$) of IL-2R+ cells were found in MS patients compared to NID.

(4) T4+2H4+ and T8+2H4+ CSF cell subsets in MS patients compared to OND (Table 3): in considering the absolute number of double marked cells, we did not find differences in T4+2H4+ and T8+2H4+ subsets, while we found a significant decrease in these subsets considered as a percentage of total T4+ cells.

(5) T4+4B4+ and T8+4B4+ CSF cell subsets in MS patients compared to OND (Table 4): in considering the absolute number of double-marked cells, significantly increased percentages ($p<0.005$) of both subsets were found. No variations in these subsets considered as a percentage of the number of T4+ and T8+ cells were observed.

DISCUSSION

As far as CSF cell subsets in MS patients are concerned (Table 1), our data confirm that the predominant cell type in MS CSF is the T lymphocyte bearing T4 marker, as reported in other studies.[11-14] Nevertheless, it is not clear if the high percentage of T4+ cells reflects a true increase in cells bearing this phenotype or if it is merely due to the decreased percentage of T8+ cells. If this increase were numerically absolute, then we could hypothesize a selective passage of T4+ cells from the blood-brain barrier to CSF. Since cytolitic T4+ clones have been isolated from MS patients,[15] T4+ subset may play an important role in nervous tissue damage. Interestingly, the T4+ cell pattern observed in ID was very different from MS (Table 1), suggesting that the T helper/inducer subset is not involved in inflammatory diseases other than MS.

Concerning the evaluation of activated cells (DR- and IL-2 receptor-bearing cells), it is known that the expression of these two molecules occurs at different times, since IL-2 R is expressed during the early stage of the activation process,[16] while DR molecule appears in the late activation phase.[17] DR+ cells in CSF are practically only T lymphocytes, since B cells and macrophages are virtually absent in CSF. Two color fluorescence cytofluorometric analysis showed that DR+ CSF cells also carried T3 phenotype (Table 5).

Several studies reported that the percentage of IL-2R-positive cells from MS in PB is higher during acute relapse than in remission,[18] or higher in CSF than in PB.[19,20] In addition, a prolonged expression of IL-2R has been reported in both antigen- or mitogen-induced T-cell lines and clones from PB and CSF of

Table 5. Percentages of cerebrospinal fluid T3+ and DR+ cells, and of DR+ cells provided by T3 receptor (T3+DR+/DR+) in multiple sclerosis (MS) and non immunological diseases of the central nervous system (NID)

	T3+	T3+DR+/T3	DR+
MS			
1	71.9	66.7	14.1
2	43.2	40.0	13.5
3	83.3	80.2	19.2
4	56.3	42.9	21.9
5	64.4	53.8	22.1
OND			
1	62.9	0.0	8.6
2	68.6	5.0	22.1

MS patients,[21] while Fredrikson et al[22] found a high percentage of DR+ CSF cells only in 10% of MS patients. In our MS patients an increase of IL-2+ cells were found compared to NID (Table 2), suggesting the presence of an antigenic stimulus in CNS; however, the slightly increased percentage of DR+ cells found in MS suggests an aberrant antigen presentation in CNS, as reported in other human diseases.[23] Alternatively, these data could indicate a selective passage of activated cells after previous contact with a peripheric antigen, as demonstrated in experimental allergic encephalomyelitis.[24]

Regarding 2H4 and 4B4 markers, Morimoto et al reported that T4+2H4+ subset is functionally characterized by the ability to induce suppression of B cell differentiation in Ig-producing cells,[9] while T4+4B4+ subset is characterized by helper-inducing function in Ig production.[10] Other studies[24,25] demonstrate that 2H4 cells are an immature stage of post-thymic differentiation culminating in 4B4 expression on cell membrane; thus Sanders et al[26] interpret 2H4 (called also CD45R) as a marker of memory cells. Several lines of investigation reported a defect in T4+2H4+ subset in PB of active[27] or progressive[28] MS patients; Rose et al[27] found the decreased 2H4 expression not only in T4+ subset but also in T8+ cells, even if this defect was found not only in MS but in other neurological diseases as well. Further on, a scarce 2H4 presence in MS lesions suggested a primary defect in 2H4 expression.[29] An opposite point of view has been formulated by Sanders et al,[30] suggesting that the loss of 2H4 marker is related to cell stimulation triggered by exogenous antigen(s): in this light, the decreased 2H4 expression in MS may be a consequence rather than a primary defect. Our data seem to confirm Sander's opinion, since we found an absolute increase in T4+4B4+ and T8+4B4+ subsets with a relative decrease in T4+2H4+ and T8+2H4+ cells. From our data, we can deduce that a selective enrichment in memory cells is present in the CSF of MS patients. Similar pattern has been reported in tubercoloid leprosy[31] and may reflect a shift from naive to memory cells at the sites of exogenous antigen exposition.

In conclusion, the imbalance in CSF lymphocytes in MS is certain, but the exact role of this imbalance in the pathogenetic mechanism of the disease is still to be clarified. The most striking data seem to be the presence in CSF of (1) a high T4/T8 ratio, (2) a small but significantly increased percentage of activated cells, and (3) a significant increase in T memory cells.

ACKNOWLEDGEMENTS

Partly supported by grants of the Italian Ministero della Pubblica Istruzione and of Regione Autonoma Sardegna.

REFERENCES

1. U. Traugott, E.L. Reinherz, C.S. Raine, Multiple sclerosis. Distribution of T cells, T cell subsets and Ia-positive macrophages in lesions of different ages, *J.Neuroimmunol.*, 4:201-221 (1983a).
2. J. Boos, M.M. Esiri, W.W. Tourtellotte, D.Y. Mason, Immunohistological analysis of T lymphocyte subsets in the central nervous system in chronic progressive multiple sclerosis, *J.Neurol.Sci.*, 62:219-232 (1983).
3. M. N. Woodroffe, A.S. Bellamy, M. Feldmann, A.B. Davison, M.L. Cuzner, Immunocytochemical characterisation of the immune reaction in the central nervous system in multiple sclerosis, *J.Neurol.Sci.*, 74:135-152 (1986).
4. H. Wekerle, C. Linington, H. Lassman, R. Meyermann, Cellular immune reactivity within the CNS, *Trends Neurosci*, 9:271-277 (1986).
5. P. E. Manconi, M.G. Marrosu, C. Cianchetti, M.G. Ennas, A. Mangoni, D. Zaccheo, Lymphocyte subpopulations in cerebrospinal fluid and peripheral blood in multiple sclerosis, *Acta Neurol.Scand.*, 62:165-175 (1980).
6. M. G. Marrosu, M.G. Ennas, M.R. Murru, G. Marrosu, C. Cianchetti, P.E. Manconi, Surface markers on lymphocytes from human cerebrospinal fluid. III. Identification by monoclonal antibodies, *J.Neuroimmunol*, 5:325-331 (1983).
7. M. G. Marrosu, C. Cianchetti, M.G. Ennas, Cerebrospinal fluid lymphocyte subpopulations in multiple sclerosis, *Ital.J.Neurol.Sci.*, 7:101-105 (1986).
8. A. S. Rose, G.W. Ellison, L.M. Myers, W.W. Tourtellotte, Criteria for the clinical diagnosis of multiple sclerosis, *Neurology*, 26:(suppl. June): 20-22 (1976).
9. C. Morimoto, N.L. Letvin, J.A. Distase, W. R. Aldrich, S.F. Schlossman, The isolation and characterization of the human suppressor inducer T cell subset, *J.Immunol.*, 134:1508-1515 (1985).
10. C. Morimoto, N.L. Letvin, A.W. Boyd, M. Hagan, H.M. Brown, M.N. Kornacki, S.F. Schlossman, The isolation and characterization of the human helper inducer T cell subset, *J.Immunol.*, 134:3762-3769 (1985).
11. N. Cashman, C. Martin, J.-F. Eizenbaum, J.-D. Degas, Monoclonal antibody defined immunoregulatory cells in multiple sclerosis cerebrospinal fluid, *J.Clin.Invest.*, 70:387-392 (1982).
12. S. L. Hauser, E.L. Weiner, CSF cells in multiple sclerosis: monoclonal antibody analysis and relationship to peripheral blood T-cell subsets, *Neurology* 33: 575-579 (1983).
13. J. Oger, J.P. Antel, A. Noronha, B.G.W. Arnason, Changes in T cell subpopulations in the cerebrospinal fluid of multiple sclerosis patients, *Neurology* 32 (suppl.2):A 148 (1982).
14. A. Noronha, D.P. Richman, B.G.W. Arnason, Multiple sclerosis: activated cells in cerebrospinal fluid in acute exacerbations, *Ann.Neurol.*, 18:722-725 (1985).
15. W. E. J. Weber, W.A. Buurman, Myelin basic protein-specific CD4+ cytolitic T-lymphocyte clones isolated from multiple sclerosis patients, *Human Immunol.*, 22:97-109.
16. D. A. Cantrell, K.A. Smith, The interleukin-2 T-cell system: a new cell growth model, *Science* 224: 1312-1316 (1984).
17. T. Cotner, J.M. Williams, L. Christenson, H.M. Shapiro, T.B. Strom, J. Strominger, Simultaneous flow cytometric analysis of human T cell activation antigen expression and DNA content, *J.Exp.Med.*, 157:461-472 (1983).
18. K. Selmaj, C. Plater-Zyberk, K.A. Rockett, R.N. Maini, R. Alam, G.D. Perkin, F. Clifford Rose, Multiple sclerosis: increased expression of interleukin-2 receptors on lymphocytes, *Neurology*, 36:1392-1395 (1986).
19. A. S. Bellamy, V.L. Calder, M. Feldmann, A.N. Davison, The distribution of interleukin-2 receptor bearing lymphocytes in multiple sclerosis:

evidence for a key role of activated lymphocytes, *Clin.Exp.Immunol.* 61:248-256 (1985).

20. E. Tournier-Lasserve, O. Lyoncaen, E. Roullet, M.A. Bach. IL-2 receptor and HLA class II antigens on cerebrospinal fluid cells of patients with multiple sclerosis and other neurological diseases, *Clin.Exp.Immunol.*, 67:581-586 (1987).
21. E. C. De Freitas, M. Sandhberg-Wollheim, K. Schonely, M. Boufal, H. Koprowski, Regulation of interleukin 2 receptors on T cells from multiple sclerosis patients, *Proc.Natl.Acad.Sci.* USA, 83:2637-2641 (1986).
22. S. Fredrikson, A.Karlsson-Parra, T. Olsson, H. Link, HLA-DR antigen expression on T cells from cerebrospinal fluid in multiple sclerosis and aseptic meningo-encephalitis, *Clin.Exp.Immunol.* 68:298-304 (1987).
23. G. F. Bottazzo, Puja-Borrell, T. Hanafusa, M. Feldmann, Role of aberrant HLA-DR expression and antigen presentation in induction of endocrine autoimmunity, *Lancet*, 2:1115-1119 (1983).
24. H. M. Serra, J.F. Krowka, J.A. Ledbetter, L.M. Pilarski, Loss of CD45R (Lp220) represents a post-thymic T cell differentiation event, *J.Immunol.*, 140:1435-1441 (1988).
25. M. E. Sanders, M.W. Makgoba, S.O. Sharrow, D. Stephany, T.M. Springer, H.A. Young, S. Shaw, Human memory T lymphocytes express increased levels of three cell adhesion molecules (LFA-3, CD2, and LFA-1) and three other molecules (UCHL1, CDw29, and PgP-1) and have enhanced IFN production, *J.Immunol.*, 140:1401-1407 (1988).
26. M. E. Sanders, M.W. Makgoba, S. Shaw, Human naive and memory T cells: reinterpretation of helper-inducer and suppressor-inducer subsets, *Immunol.Today*, 9:195-199 (1988).
27. L. M. Rose, A.H. Ginsberg, T.L. Rothstein, J.A. Ledbetter, E.A. Clark, Selective loss of a subset of T helper cells in active multiple sclerosis, *Proc.Natl.Acad.Sci.* USA 82:7389-7393 (1985).
28. C. Morimoto, D.A. Hafler, H.L. Weiner, N.L. Letvin, M. Hagain, J. Daley, S.F. Schlossman, Selective loss of the suppressor-inducer T cell subset in progressive multiple sclerosis, *N.Engl.J.Med.* 316:67-72 (1987).
29. R. A. Sobel, D.A. Hafler, E.E. Castro, C. Morimoto, H.L. Weiner, The 2H4 (CD45R) antigen is selectively decreased in multiple sclerosis lesions, *J.Immunol.*, 140:2210-2214 (1988).
30. M. E. Sanders, M.W. Makgoba, S. Shaw, Alterations in T cell subsets in multiple sclerosis and other autoimmune diseases, *Lancet* 2: 1021-1021 (1988).
31. R. L.Modlin, J. Melancon-Kaplan, S.M.M. Young, C. Pirmez, H. Kino, J. Convit, T. H. Rea, B.R. Bloom, Learning from lesions: patterns of tissue inflammation in leprosy, *Proc.Natl.Acad.Sci.* USA 85:1213-1217 (1988).

FUNCTIONAL CHARACTERISTICS AND PHENOTYPIC MARKERS OF T LYMPHOCYTE CLONES FROM CSF IN MULTIPLE SCLEROSIS

V. Barnaba, R. Benvenuto, C. Buttinelli*, A. Franco, S. Bernardi*, M.G. Grasso*, F. Balsano, and C. Fieschi*

I Medical Clinic, University of Rome, and
*Department of Neurological Sciences, University of Rome
Rome, Italy

INTRODUCTION

Multiple sclerosis (MS) is a chronic, inflammatory, demyelinating disease of the central nervous system (CNS),[1,2] characterized by infiltrating cells, predominantly T cells,[3,4] in the sites of active demyelinization. In the cerebrospinal fluid (CSF), the majority of cells are CD4 T lymphocytes,[5,6] while CD8 T cells are depressed during the acute phases, as well as in peripheral blood. Functional studies of CSF lymphocytes were hampered by the small number of cells available after lumbar puncture. In this study we established cloned T cell lines from the CSF of one MS patient to investigate their phenotype and functional capacities.

MATERIALS AND METHODS

Patient

One female, aged 30 years, with clinically definite MS (according to Schumacher criteria[7]) and relapsing-progressive disease was studied. She was followed at the Department of Neurological Sciences of Rome. The patient was not treated with immunosuppressive therapy for at least 6 months before the study. CSF cells were obtained during exacerbation phase of the disease.

Immunological assays

Isolation of lymphocytes. CSF was obtained through lumbar puncture and immediately centrifuged at 1200 rpm at 4°C. The cells were washed in RPMI 1640 (Flow Lab. UK) supplemented with 10% heat inactivated FCS (Flow Lab. UK), 1% Glutamine (Flow Laboratories, 25 mM Hepes (Gibco), 1% sodium pyruvate (Flow Lab), 100 U/ml Penicillin (Flow Lab), 100 -µg/ml Streptomycin (Flow Lab), and 2.5 µg/ml Fungizone (Flow Lab) (complete medium).

Generation of CSF-derived T cell clones. CSF lymphocytes were immediately cloned by limiting dilution at 1 cell/well in the presence of 1 µg/ml Phytoemoagglutinin (PHA), 105 allogeneic irradiated peripheral blood mononuclear cells(iPEMC) and 50 U/ml rIL2 (Biogen). After 2 weeks, cell growth was detected using an inverted microscope. The growing cells were expanded further in medium with PHA, allogeneic iPEMC and IL2 every 2-3 weeks.

Table 1. Cell Surface Phenotype of 46 CSF T Cell Clones

No. of clones	CD3	CD4	CD8	WT31
40	98%	98%	2%	98%
6	98%	2%	98%	98%

Table 2. LDCC* and NK† Cytolytic Activities of CSF T Cell Clones

CSF Clone	Phenotype	LDCC (%) Without PHA	LDCC (%) With PHA	NK (%)
A2	CD8	32.7	82.2	33.3
D5	CD8	7.1	73.4	62.4
E4	CD8	6.24	28.9	55.2
E12	CD8	10.1	95.8	76.6
F11	CD8	4.2	122.0	88.4
G5	CD8	12.4	69.5	91.1
A1	CD4	7.4	27.7	1
A3	CD4	29.3	70.6	4.3
C8	CD4	15.5	39.8	1.2
C9	CD4	1	21.6	2.6
C10	CD4	2	17.4	5
C11	CD4	2	15.8	1
C12	CD4	3.4	13.5	4.6
D7	CD4	6.5	13.5	nd
D8	CD4	2.1	1.1	7.66
D9	CD4	1.7	8.8	nd
E3	CD4	4.9	5.2	7.8
E5	CD4	1	15.0	1
E8	CD4	1	22.5	1
F3	CD4	3.8	19.9	11.59
F4	CD4	1	7.4	nd
F5	CD4	1	10.2	1
G1	CD4	1	14.8	4.7
G3	CD4	9.9	5.5	nd
G4	CD4	1	21.0	1
G8	CD4	1	18.0	nd

* LDCC activity of T clones in a 4-hr ^{51}Cr-release assay against an NK-resistant murine P815 cell line at an E/T ratio of 10:1.
† NK activity of T clones in a 4-hr ^{51}Cr-release assay against an NK-sensitive human K562 cell line at an E/T ratio of 10:1.
nd = Not determined.

Surface phenotypic analysis. The surface phenotype of CSF derived T-cell clones was determined by indirect immunofluorescence microscopy using murine monoclonal antibodies: OKT3, OKT4, OKT8, OKDR, OKT26a (Ortho, Raritan, NY), antiTCR1(WT31) (Becton Dickinson Mountain View, CA).

Cytotoxic function. Cytotoxic T lymphocytes (CTL) activity was tested in a 4-hr ^{51}Cr release assay. Cloned T cells, used a effector cells were incubated into the U bottomed wells of microtiter trays (Falcon) with ^{51}Cr labelled target cells at effector/target ratios of 10:1. The cell lines used as targets in cytotoxicity assays were the NK-sensitive K562 cell line (NK activity) and the NK-resistant murine

Table 3. Helper Activity of CSF T Cell Clones on PWM-driven Ig by Allogeneic PBL*

CSF Clone	Phenotype	IgG (ng/ml)	IgM (ng/ml)
-	-	1785	721
A1	CD4	1522	700
A3	CD4	95	84
C8	CD4	1602	643
C10	CD4	10713	4500
D8	CD4	3482	1462
D9	CD4	54635	2173
E3	CD4	8933	3605
F4	CD4	7144	2884
F5	CD4	12443	5005
G3	CD4	3566	2333

*PBL were cultured with or without various T clones in the presence of PWM (1/100 vol/vol) for 10 days. Supernatants were assayed for Ig by ELISA.

P815 cell line in the presence of 1 μg/ml PHA (Lectin dependent cell mediated cytotoxicity; LDCC), that detects cytolytic T lymphocytes irrespective of their-specificity. Microplates were centrifuged and 0.1 ml supernatants (SN) was assayed for ^{51}Cr release. The specific lysis was calculated as percentage cytotoxicity according to the formula: (experimental release - spontaneous release/ total release - spontaneous release) x 100.

Antigen specificity. T cell clones were tested for their proliferative response to Myelin basic protein (MEP). The proliferative response was measured by the incorporation of [^{3}H]-thymidine into DNA by replicate cultures. Results are expressed as mean cpm of the replicates.

Helper activity. Peripheral blood lymphocytes (PBL) were cultured with or without various T cell clones in the presence of pokeweed mitogen (PWM) (1:100 vol/vol) for 10 days. Supernatants were assayed for Ig by ELISA.

RESULTS AND DISCUSSION

Forty six cell clones were generated and studied for their phenotype and functional capacity: 40 clones were CD4+ and six were CD8+ (Table 1). All resulted DR+, TAC+ and expressed alpha/beta heterodimer of the antigen T cell receptor (WT31). None out of ten CSF clones tested (eight CD4 and two CD8) showed any reactivity to myelin basic protein. All the CD8 clones expressed NK-like function and CTL activity assessed by an LDCC assay detecting cytolitic potential of T cells irrespective of their specificity (Table 2) suggesting a selective accumulation of cytotoxic precursor CD8 cells in CSF. In contrast only six out of 20 CD4 clones displayed CTL function; these cytotoxic CD4 clones lacked NK function. It is not surprising that in addition T clones with CD4 phenotypic, that are considered define T 'helper cells', act as cytotoxic cells. Recently it has been demonstrated that not all cytotoxic T cells are restricted by class I MHC determinants, but that class II restricted cytolysis may be important in normal anti-viral immune reactivity.[8] Seven out of ten CD4 clones, tested for their ability to modulate PWM-induced Ig responses by normal allogeneic PBL, strongly enhanced the polyclonal response (Table 3); the three CD4 clones lacking helper function showed cytotoxic activity, suggesting that the true helper T cells lack cytotoxic activity and therefore, B cells and antigen presenting cells will not be killed during antigen presentation.

These clones would be extremely useful in testing the specificity and the cytotoxic function of the CSF clones against different viral antigens or targets infected with a variety of viruses, in order to identify a possible virus involved in the disease. Furthermore, the analysis of T cells in the CSF of MS patients at the clonal level could be used to investigate their antigen receptor gene rearrangements.

REFERENCES

1. B. H. Waksman and W.E. Reynolds, Multiple sclerosis as a disease of immune regulation, *Proc.Soc.Exp.Biol.Med.*USA, 175:282 (1984).
2. H. L. Weiner and D.A. Hafler, Multiple sclerosis, *in:* "Current Neurology," S. Appel, ed., Vol.6, p.123 (1986).
3. U. Traugott, E.L. Reinherz, and C.S. Raine, Multiple sclerosis: distribution of T cell subsets with active chronic lesions, *Science*, 219:308 (1983).
4. S. L. Hauser, A.K. Bhan, F. Gilles, M. Kemp, C. Karr, and H.L. Weiner, Immunohistochemical analysis of the cellular infiltrate in multiple sclerosis lesions, *Ann.Neurol.*, 19:578 (1986).
5. N. Cashman, C. Martin, J.F. Eizenbaum, J.D. Degos, and M.A. Bach, Monoclonal antibody-defined immunoregulatory cells in multiple sclerosis cerebrospinal fluid, *J.Clin.Invest.*, 70:387 (1982).
6. M. Sandberg-Wollheim, M. Lymphocyte, Population in the cerebrospinal fluid and peripheral blood of patients with multiple sclerosis and optic neuritis, *Scand.J.Immunol.*, 17:757 (1983).
7. G. A. Schumacher, G. Beebe, R.F. Kibler, L.T. Kurland, J.F. Kurtzke, F. McDowell, B.Nager, W.A. Sibley, W. Tourtelotte, T.L. Wilmont, Problems of experimental trials of therapy in multiple sclerosis: report by the panel on the evaluation of experimental trials of therapy of multiple sclerosis, *Ann.Ny.Acad.Sci.*, 122:552-568 (1965).
8. S. J. Jacobson, J.R. Richert, W.E. Biddison, A. Satinsky, R.J. Hartzman, H.F. McFarland, Measles virus-specific T4+ human cytotoxic T cell clones are restricted by class II HLA antigens, *J.Immunol.*, 133:754 (1984).

MULTIPLE SCLEROSIS: LYMPHOCYTE RESPONSES TO CNS ANTIGENS

V. L. Calder, S. J. Owen and A. N. Davison

Department of Neurochemistry
Institute of Neurology
Queen Square, London WC1N 3BG, U. K.

INTRODUCTION

In multiple sclerosis (MS), T lymphocytes are observed in the perivascular cuffs[1] and increased numbers of activated T cells are detected in cerebrospinal fluid (CSF) samples from some MS patients,[2] suggesting an ongoing immune response. T cells are clearly involved in experimental allergic encephalomyelitis (EAE) for demyelinating disease can be induced in SJL mice after adoptively transferring cloned T cells reactive to the encephalitogenic region of myelin basic protein.[3] Thus a role for T cells in the pathogenesis of MS has been proposed. Although the origin and specificity of these autoimmune T cells remains obscure, recent reports suggest that $CD2^+$ T cells rapidly migrate from the peripheral blood into the central nervous system (CNS).[4] The peripheral blood might therefore be useful for monitoring the ongoing pathological process within the CNS.

In order to test this hypothesis we have examined the proliferative responses of peripheral blood lymphocytes (PBL) from MS, other neurological diseases (OND) and healthy controls to two CNS antigens - myeling basic protein (MBP) and brain gangliosides. Responses to synthetic peptides of MBP were also studied. We found significant responses to all CNS antigens under test which did not correlate with the clinical stage of disease. The possible reasons for this finding are discussed.

MATERIALS AND METHODS

Patients

All patients had definite MS, according to the criteria of McDonald and Halliday[5]. Patients were classified as in relapse when a new clinical sign had developed within the last 3 weeks. Patients with active disease had a clear previous history of new signs or symptoms within the last 3 months. Progressive cases of MS had evidence of lesions at two or more separate sites in the CNS and also a history of progressive paraplegia. None of the patients or controls were receiving immunosuppressive therapy. Patients with OND included epilepsy, brainstem stroke and Guillain-Barré syndrome.

Peripheral Blood Lymphocytes

Whole heparinized blood was diluted 1:1 in fetal calf serum-containing medium (FCS-RPMI) and layered over Ficoll-Hypaque at 1000 g for 15 min. After washing, cells were resuspended in RPMI 1640 containing 10% FCS, penicillin/streptomycin and 2 mM L-glutamine.

Proliferation Assay

PBL were plated out in triplicate at $2x10^5$ cells per well in 96-well flat bottom tissue culture plates at 37°C, 5% CO_2 in the presence of antigen at a range of concentrations (50-0.001 μg/ml). Each well was pulsed with 1°Ci ^{3}H-thymidine on the fifth day for 8 hr prior to harvesting and counting in a scintillation counter. Mean counts per minute (cpm) were calculated for each triplicate and scored as positive when counts were greater than or equal to twice those of control wells (cells without antigen). A response to the mitogen phytohaemagglutinin (PHA; 1 μg/ml) was always included as a positive control The stimulation index (SI) was thus calculated as:

$$SI = \text{mean cpm} \quad \frac{\text{(cells with antigen).}}{\text{(cells alone)}}$$

Antigens

Human myelin basic protein (MBP) was generously provided by Dr P. Glynn (Institute of Neurology, London, UK) and was prepared as described by Dunkley and Carnegia.[6] Mixed bovine brain gangliosides were a gift from Fidia Laboratories, Milan, Italy. Phytohaemagglutinin (PHA) was obtained from Difco Laboratories, UK. Synthetic peptides of human MBP were kindly provided by Dr N. Groome (Oxford, UK).[7]

RESULTS

Responses to MBP and Gangliosides

A total of 61 MS cases were examined for their response to MBP and gangliosides (see Table 1). A significant response (SI≥2) to either of the antigens was observed in 27/61 (44%) MS cases in comparison with 3/12 (25%) OND and 4/11 (36%) healthy. No significant difference in the response to PHA was

Table 1. Response of MS Peripheral Blood Lymphocytes to Synthetic Peptides of Myelin Basic Protein (MBP) in Comp[arison with Whole MBP

MS Patients	Stikulation Index for response to MBP	Peptides
I	2	2 (P10, P20, P21, P27)
II	2	2 (P21, P27)
III	1	2 (P10)
IV	1	2 (P21)
V	1	7 (P16)
		2 (P20)
VI	1	2 (P13)

Peptide sequences tested: P13 (position 36-50); P20 (51-64); P27 (61-75); P16 (64-78); P21 (69-83); P10 (75-89); P12 (80-97); P15 (91-106).

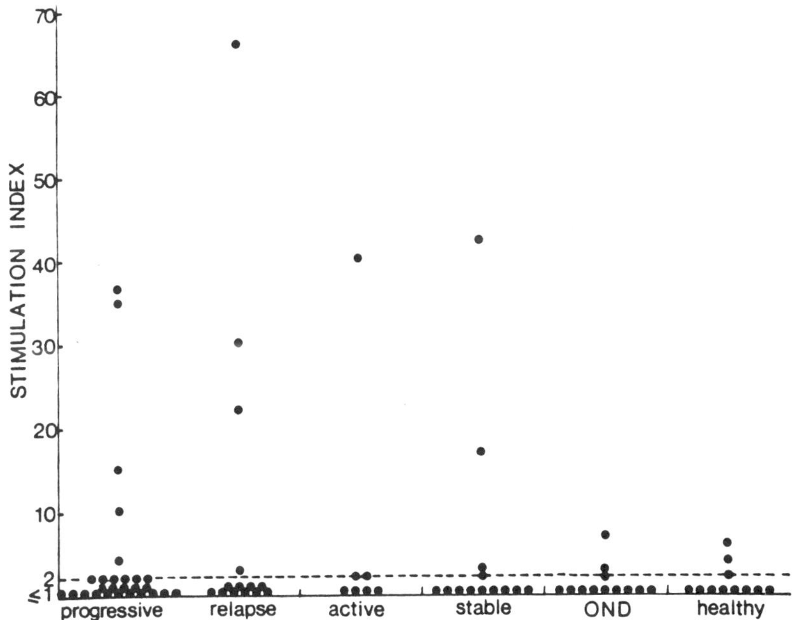

Fig. 1. Comparison of the stimulation index of responses to MBP by PBL from MS (progressive, relapse, active, stable), OND and healthy cases. A positive response to MBP is where SI≥2.

observed between the groups. The optimum antigen concentrations were found to be: MBP (O.O1-10 µg/ml); gangliosides (0.001-0.1 µg/ml).

Comparison of SI Values

The stimulation index (SI) of each response was plotted for each separate group (see Fig. 1). Calculating mean ±SEM for the response to MBP, progressive MS was 4.8 (1.8), relapse 9.36 (4.99), active 6.86 (5.53) and stable MS 5.69 (3.26). In the control groups, OND were 1.75 (=.5) and healthy cases were 1.8 (=.5). Using the *F*-test to compare variability between sample means, all MS groups showed statistically significant variability in response to MBP in comparison with OND and healthy cases. Similarly for response to gangliosides, progressive MS cases had mean SI values of 4.33 (2.0), relapse 8.85 (4.39), active 18.43 (16.9) and stable MS 1.92 (0.46). These SI values showed a significant increase in variability in comparison with than OND cases 1.75 (0.46) and healthy controls 1.9 (0.5).

Responses to Synthetic BP Peptides:

Since there could be a low level contamination of our MBP preparation, we examined 17 MS cases for responses to MBP and to synthetic short peptide sequences in the encephalitogenic region of the human MBP molecule.[7] Low but significant responses to the peptide sequences were observed in 6 of the cases examined where SI ≥2. Peptides were tested over a wide range of concentrations and were found to give responses at a final concentration of 0.01-10 µg/ml (see Table 1).

DISCUSSION

Evidence for the reactivity of T lymphocytes to the myelin antigen MBP has been a matter of controversy since the early studies showing cell mediated hypersensitivity to MBP by cell migration assay.[8] Inconclusive data has also bee reported using the classical lymphocyte transformation assay with MBP as antigen[9]. A number of factors might account for the variable responses of PBL in MS found by different investigators. In some studies high concentrations of MBP were used in the assay which suppress rather than stimulate the antigen response. Secondly the purity of different MBP preparations varies and deteriorates on storage. In addition the number of MBP-reactive T cells in blood is small. When very low concentrations of MBP are used in the lymphocyte transformation assay we have been able to detect significant responses to MBP and to MBP peptides in the PBL of a few MS patients. Such responses do not correlate with the clinical status of the patients. Similarly, responses to brain gangliosides were found at low concentrations (ng/ml) and no correlation with disease status was seen. However recent MRI studies demonstrating the appearance of new lesions in the absence of any clinical signs might explain the lack of correlation we have found in our results.

Evidence from the literature[10] and our own published suggests that MBP-sensitized cells may be more abundant in the CSF than in the blood. We have therefore proposed that the inflammatory reaction is initiated within the CNS and that the autoaggressive cells spill over from the CSF into the periphery. However the role of MBP-sensitized T cells in central demyelination is so far unknown. It has recently been shown that MBP induces release of lymphokines including tumour necrosis factor by T lymphocytes from MS patients.[11] These lymphocytes may thus mediate myeling damage or recruit other cells from the peripheral blood into the CNS to form the characteristic perivascular inflammatory cuffs seen in acute lesions. Another possibility is that sensitization of lymphocytes to CNS antigens is a secondary phenomenon. However the demonstration that MBP-specific rodent T cells can induce demyelination both in tissue culture[12] and in isolated myelin preparations[13] suggests that the MBP-specific T lymphocyte is functionally involved in primary demyelination.

REFERENCES

1. V. Traugott, E.L. Reinhert, C. S. Raine, J.Neuroimmunol., 4:201 (1983).
2. A S. Bellamy, V.L. Calder, M. Feldmann, A.N. Davison, *Clin.Exp.Imm.*, 61:248-256 (1985).
3. S. Zamvil, P. Nelson, J. Trotter, D. Mitchell, R. Knobler, R. Fritz, L. Steinman, *Nature,* 317:355-358 (1985).
4. D. A. Hafler, H.L. Winer, *Ann.Neurol.*, 22:89-93 (1987).
5. W. I. McDonald, A.N. Halliday, *Brit.Med.Bull.*, 33:4-8 (1977).
6. P. R. Dunkley, P.R. Carnegie, Isolation of myelin basic protein, *in:* 'Research Methods in Neurochemistry,' vol. 2, W. Marks and R. Rodnight, ed., Plenum Press, N.Y. (1977).
7. N. Groome, et al., J.Neuroimm, (in press) (1988).
8. S. P. Colby, W. Sheremata, B. Bain, E. Eylar, *Neurol,* 21;132:139 (1977).
9. R A.C. Hughes, L. A. Gray, R. Clifford-Jones, M. A. Stern, *Acta Neurol.Scand.* 60:65-76 (1979).
10. R P. Lisak, B. Zinerman, *New Engl.J.Med.*, 297:850-853 (1977).
11. C S.Brosnan, K. Selmaj, C. S. Raine, *J.Neuroimm,* 18:87-94 (1988).
12. W. D. Lyman, G.A. Roth, C.F. Brosnan, M.B. Bornstein, C.S. Raine, *J.Neuroimm* 17:175-180 (1988).
13. C M. Watson, J. Najbauer, S.J. Owen, A.N. Davison, *J.Neurochem.*, 50:1469-1477 (1988).

Immune Functions of Glia

IMMUNOREGULATION IN THE CENTRAL NERVOUS SYSTEM: DETECTION OF CYTOKINES IN CEREBROSPINAL FLUID

A. Fontana, K. Frei, P. Gallo, T.P. Leist, D. Leppert, U.V. Malipiero and D. Nadal

Section of Clinical Immunology, University Hospital
Haeldeliweg 4, CH-8044 Zürich, Switzerland

INTRODUCTION

To initiate an immune response after recognition of antigen presented in the context of class II antigens of the major histocompatibility complex (MHC) on macrophages, dendritic cells or B cells, T helper cells become activated. This process involves direct cell-cell contact mediated by adhesion reactions, eg, between the lymphocyte function-associated antigen-one (LFA-1) on T cells and its ligand, the intercellular adhesion molecule-1 (ICAM-1) on antigen presenter cells. This allows the triggering of the T cells by binding of antigen to the T cell antigen receptor/CD3 complex which transduces antigen-specific extracellular stimuli across the plasma membrane, generating intracellular signals. These events render T cells competent to receive progression signals to enter from G_1 the S phase, a process mediated by interleukin-2 binding to its receptor. In addition to direct cell-cell contacts, soluble factors released by lymphocytes, monocytes-macrophages or by cells not belonging to the immune system (eg, keratinocytes or fibroblasts) are also involved in the maturation, growth and activation of the cellular elements of the immune system. Provided their synthesis by parenchymal cells of different organs, cytokines, polypeptide mediators that transmit signals from one cell to another, may propagate local expansion and activation of lymphocytes having infiltrated the tissue through the vessel wall. In the brain, T cell infiltrates can be observed mainly in viral diseases and multiple sclerosis. Besides T cells, there is evidence also that monocytes and B cells invade the brain parenchyma and/or the meninges. The hypothesis of intracerebral immune regulatory signals acting on infiltrating T and B cells is substantiated by the finding of (1) inducible expression of MHC class I and II antigens on astrocytes and microglial cells (reviewed in reference [1], (2) the demonstration of cytokines released by glial cells *in vivo* and (3) the detection of cytokines in the cerebrospinal fluid (CSF) of patients with immune mediated brain diseases or experimental animals with infectious diseases of the central nervous system (CNS).

In this review, we describe the recent demonstration of tumor necrosis factor α (TNFα), interferon-γ(IFNγ), interleukin-6 (IL-6)/B cell stimulatory factor-2 (BSF-2) and interleukin-1 (IL-1) in the CSF in inflammatory diseases of the CNS.

INTERFERON γ IN VIRAL DISEASES OF THE BRAIN

IFNγ has many of the antiviral, antiproliferative and immunomodulatory functions of other types of interferon. However, IFNγ is unique in its ability to induce class II MHC antigens on, for example, monocytes enabling these cells to function as antigen presenter cells. In the CNS, cells bearing MHC class II antigens (Ia/DR) are underrepresented compared to other organs. However, IFNγ injected directly into the brain of mice or added to cultured murine brain cells in vitro triggers the expression of Ia antigens on astrocytes and microglial cells. In experimental allergic encephalitis, as well as in multiple sclerosis, microglial cells/brain macrophages in addition to infiltrating monocytes but also some astrocytes have been identified as being Ia positive. The expression of Ia antigens may be triggered by infiltrating preactivated T helper cells type one, or by cytotoxic T cells, which release IFNγ in the tissue. However, as recently coronavirus was found to induce Ia antigens on astrocytes, IFNγ independent mechanisms triggered by virus directly may also give rise to Ia positive cells (for review see reference 1).

In recent experiments we have shown that IFNγ is produced in the CNS in mice infected intracerebrally with lymphocytic choriomeningitis virus (LCMV).[2] Whereas no IFNγ (measured by radioimmunoassay) was detected in the CSF samples during the first 5 days after infection, a sharp increase of IFNγ was noted on Days 6 and 7. In contrast, serum levels of IFNγ gradually increased between Days 2 and 5. However, the levels of IFNγ were up to 1000-fold lower (Day 7) in the serum compared to CSF. This speaks in favor of IFNγ to be produced within the CNS. The sources of the IFNγ detected are very likely LCMV-specific T cells which penetrate into the CNS in the course of LCMV disease (see below). This conclusion is supported by the absence of IFNγ in CSF of LCMV infected athymic nu/nu mice which do not develop disease (see below).

Recently, the intrathecal synthesis of IFNγ in CSF of patients with herpes encephalitis has been reported.[3] The synthesis was concomitant with that of interferon α and switched off when the specific antiviral antibodies in the CSF increased. Interestingly, both acute postinfectious measles and postinfectious rubella encephalitis, as well as subacute sclerosing panecephalitis, were not paralled by measurable IFNγ production in the CNS.

Low IFNγ in CSF has also been reported in all the CSF samples of 30 multiple sclerosis patients tested. However, no CSF controls were included in the study and the amount of IFNγ was very low (0.3-1.4 U/ml).[4] In the investigation on IFNγ by Lebon et al[5] none of 27 cases of multiple sclerosis was detected to be positive for IFNγ - levels of 0.3 U/ml were found not to be IFNγ specific. Taken together, these data provide evidence for intrathecal synthesis of IFNγ in immune mediated diseases, the IFNγ being produced may not only turn on facultative antigen presenting cells to fulfill their function but may also regulate the intracerebral immune response (eg, to enhance production of antiviral antibodies by infiltrating B cells).

INTRATHECAL SYNTHESIS OF B CELLS STIMULATORY FACTOR 2/INTERLEUKIN 6

There is substantial evidence for B cell activation in the CNS in viral diseases. In acute or chronic viral infections or in multiple sclerosis, B lymphocytes and plasma cells can be detected in the brain tissue.[6,7] Production of

Table 1. Cytokines in CSF

Cytokine	Disease	CSF pos./total	Authors
IFNγ	Herpes simplex	14/16	Lebon et al 1988[3]
	Postinfectious encephalitis		
	- measles	0/6	
	- rubella	0/7	
	SSPE	0/7	
IFNγ	Multiple sclerosis	30/30	Hirsch et al 1985[4]
IFNγ	Multiple sclerosis	0/29	Lebon et al 1987[5]
IFNγ	Mice with acute LCMW disease	Positive*	Frei et al 1988[2]
BSF-2	Viral meningitis	25/42	Houssian et al 1988[21]
	Herpes simplex encephalitis	9/24	
	Neurolues	0/11	
	SSPE	0/5	
	Multiple sclerosis	1/30	
	Lyme disease	1/12	
	OND	0/65	
BSF-2	Viral meningitis	12/15	Frei et al 1988[2]
	Herpes simplex encephalitis	4/4	
	Multiple sclerosis	1/31	
	OND	0/16	
BSF-2	Mice with acute LCMW/VSV disease	Positive*	Frei et al 1988[2]
TNFα	Bacterial meningitis	12/17	Gallo et al 1988[28]
	Viral meningitis	0/15	
	Multiple sclerosis	0/40	
	OND	0/16	
TNFα	Mice with		
	- listeria meningitis	Positive*	Leist et al 1988[27]
	- LCMV disease	Negative	
IL-1	Degenerative spinal disease	12/13	Gorczynski & Keystone 1986[40]
IL-1	Severe head injury	12/12	McClain et al 1987[41]
	Degenerative spinal diseases	0/?	
IL-1	Guinea pigs with chronic relapsing EAE	Positive	Symons et al 1987[42]
IL-1	Cats treated with		
	- LPS, iv	Negative	Coceani et al 1988[43]
	- IL-1, iv	Negative	
	- LPS, ic	Positive	

* CSF samples of 3 - 6 mice were pooled and tested for their lymphokine activity.

immunoglobulins (Ig) within the CNS is suggested by the finding of an increased IgG/albumin ratio in CSF compared to serum and by the detection of oligoclonal bands of IgG and abnormal kappa/lambda ratios in CSF (reviewed in references 8-10). There is evidence that in viral brain diseases the IgG bands of apparently restricted specificity are directed against the etiologic agent, eg, measles virus in subacute sclerosing panecephalitis. In addition, however, in multiple sclerosis an unexplained generalized B cell stimulation with elevated CSF antibodies to multiple viruses has been described. The signals which trigger B cells in the brain tissue to undergo clonal expansion and maturation to synthesize and secrete antibodies are not known.

Recently, the cloning of cDNAs of several factors involved in activation of resting B cells, and in growth or differentiation of activated B cells has been reported.[11] A T lymphocyte derived factor named B cell stimulatory factor 2 (BSF-2) which is also known as hybridoma/plasmacytoma growth factor,[12] 26 kDa protein,[13] interferon β2 [14] or interleukin-6 [11] was found to induce the final differentiation step of B cells to high-rate Ig secretion.[11] When tested on human lymphoblastoid cell lines BSF-2 induced an increase in both μ- and γ–chain mRNA transcription specific for Ig-heavy chains.[15] Recombinant BSF-2 added to B blast cells induced synthesis of IgM, IgG and IgA. This effect could be inhibited with anti-BSF-2 antibodies.[16] Our studies demonstrate the production of BSF-2 in the CNS, a finding which may explain effective intrathecal Ig production.

In order to evaluate for BSF-2 as well as IFNγ (see above) produced intrathecally in infectious CNS diseases, mice were infected with LCMV (100 to 300 pfu) or vesicular stomatitis virus (VSV) (5×10^3 pfu). The two model infections in mice differ in their pathogenesis. Acute experimental LCMV infection which leads to death within 6 to 8 days is characterized by an inflammatory response in the leptomeninges, the ependymal layer and chorioid plexus. Many studies have implicated T cells as central to the development of LCMV disease. The presence of cytotoxic T cells (Lyt-2^+) with an almost absence of L3T4^+ cells in the CSF has been shown by flow microfluorometry.[17] The crucial role of Lyt-2^+ cells is evidenced by the induction of disease by LCMV specific Lyt-2^+ cells injected into immunosuppressed LCMV infected mice which as a result of the T cell transfer develop an acute CNS disease.[18] In contrast, infection with VSV causes an acute encephalitis due to the cytopathogenic effects on brain parenchymal cells; death occurs in both T cell deficient athymic mice as well as in normal mice within 3 - 4 days after intracerebral infection.

In the CSF, BSF-2 was measured by a bioassay using the BSF-2 dependent B cell hybridoma 7TD1. Both IFNγ and BSF-2 can only be detected in CSF of normal ICR +/+ mice with acute LCMV disease.[2] In athymic ICR nu/nu mice, which do not develop LCMV disease neither IFNγ nor BSF-2 becomes measurable in the CSF. However, unlike IFNγ - a product of activated T cells - BSF-2 was found in very high levels in the CSF of athymic nu/nu mice with acute VSV infection, the amounts of BSF-2 being up to 60 times higher in CSF compared to serum.[19] These observations suggested that in the brain, synthesis of BSF-2 may take place not only by invading T cells but also by brain parenchymal cells. Indeed, both cultured astrocytes and microglial cells of ICR +/+ mice secrete BSF-2 when infected with LCMV.[19] Fibroblasts have recently also been found to secrete BSF-2 when infected with different RNA and DNA viruses.[20] As in mice, BSF-2 has been demonstrated in two independent studies of patients with viral meningitis and viral encephalitis.[2,21]

The local production of BSF-2 by glial cells and/or by T cells/monocytes which have invaded the brain parenchyma or meninges may amplify the maturation of infiltrating virus immune B lymphocytes and activate them *in situ* to a high rate of secretion of antiviral antibodies to prevent further spread of cytopathic virus. As BSF-2 was also observed to induce synthesis of nerve growth factor (NGF) by astrocytes *in vitro*, BSF-2 production in the CNS may contribute to neurotrophic support.[19]

TUMOR NECROSIS FACTOR α AS AN INDICATOR OF BACTERIAL MENINGITIS

TNFα (for review see references 22,23) was initially discovered because of its tumor-killing activity *in vivo*. Some cultured cell lines, such as the La D98, BT-20, MCF-7 and ME-180, are highly sensitive to the cytotoxic action of TNF *in vitro*. Many others are sensitive to the toxic action only when cotreated with interferon, particularly IFNγ. It has to be pointed out that non-transformed cells remain unaffected by TNF treatment. However, when treated also with an inhibitor of transcription or protein synthesis or with interleukin-1, some of these normal diploid cells (eg, pancreatic islet cells) can also be lysed - except some transformed B cells, lymphocytes and erythrocytes nearly all cells are positive for TNF receptors. In the CNS, TNFα has been suggested to mediate macrophage induced demyelination, as TNFα had some cytotoxic activity on rat oligodendrocytes.[24] Besides causing tumor regression *in vivo*, TNFα is also a central regulator of inflammation and immunity. In the context of the finding of TNFα in the CSF in bacterial meningitis (see below), it is interesting that TNFα has direct effects on granulocytes, increasing their attachment to the vessel wall, their migration into damaged tissue and their production of toxic oxygen products that destroy bacteria. On endothelial cells, TNFα induces the secretion of procoagulant activity, the secretion of IL-1α and IL-1β and the expression of MHC class I antigens and of an adhesion molecule for lymphocytes termed RR-1. Upon injection into rats, high doses of TNFα cause hemorrhagic necrosis being indistinguishable from that resulting from endotoxin administration. Endotoxin shock and death can be prevented by antibodies against TNFα. These studies were all done with cachectin which later turned out to be identical to TNFα. By suppressing the lipoprotein lipase, cachectin/TNFα inhibits the normal storage of fact and causes cachexia (for review see references 22,23).

In vivo TNFα/cachectin was originally detected in the serum of mice infected with *Bacillus Calmette-Guerin* (BCG) and subsequently injected with endotoxin. When sera from patients with a variety of infectious diseases were examined (eg, various fungal and bacterial infections), only those from patients with visceral leishmaniasis (18 of 27 sera) or malaria (seven of 10 sera) showed a raised frequency of elevated TNFα levels.[25] Of 79 serum samples tested of patients with meningococcal disease, 18 contained TNFα.[26] In the group of patients with meningococcal meningitis, only four of the 41 sera were positive. In previous investigations we have searched for TNFα in CSF and serum of animals with experimental infectious meningitis or patients with acute meningitis.

C57BL/6 mice which were infected intracerebrally with listeria monocytogenes (600 cfu) died between Days 3 and 4 after infection. The CSF showed marked pleocytosis with predominantly polymorphonuclear cells (>90%). In the brain an intense meningitis was observed. Already 3 hr after infection TNFα was detected in the CSF; the levels further increased over the next 24 - 48 hr.[27] Interestingly, TNFα was not detected in the serum of these mice suggesting intrathecal synthesis of TNFα Furthermore, TNFα was also not observed in mice infected with LCMV - this was even true prior to death of the animals (Day 6 to Day 7).[27] Thus, bacterial meningitis was distinguishable from viral meningitis on the basis of the occurrence of TNFα in CSF. By in situ hybridization using an antisense TNFα probe, however, low numbers of TNFα mRNA positive cells (3-7.7%) were identified also in the inflammatory cell infiltrate in LCMV disease.[26] Thus, the negative finding of TNFα in CSF may reflect either post-transcriptional regulation of TNFα biosynthesis or consumption of TNFα at the lesion site.

In analogy to the animal study, all samples of 12 patients with acute bacterial meningitis due to *Neisseria meningitis, Haemophilus influenzae* or *Streptococcus pneumoniae* were positive for TNFα when tested by ELISA. Of five patients who had clinically improved (after Day 3 of admission to the hospital), the CSF did not contain TNFα. TNFα was also not detected in the CSF of patients with acute aseptic viral meningitis, subacute or chronic bacterial (Treponema pallidum, Mycobacterium tuberculosis), fungous and protozoan meningitis/ meningoencephalitis.[28] The intrathecal synthesis of TNFα in bacterial meningitis may contribute to the blood-brain barrier damage observed in meningitis. Furthermore, TNFα may exert direct cytotoxic effects and/or operate by activating polymorphonuclear cells to release toxic radicals. Sensitive ELISA techniques may be of diagnostic help to evaluate for the presence of TNFα in CSF from patients with acute meningitis of unknown or uncertain ethiology.

INTERLEUKIN-1 OR INTERLEUKIN-6 IN ACUTE EAE?

IL-1 is a polypeptide synthesized by a variety of cell types including those of hematological (mainly monocytes-macrophages), dermasomal (keratinocytes) and neuronal (astrocytes, microglial cells) origin. Many of the activities attributed to TNFα are also mediated by IL-1, which is an immunomodulatory molecule that promotes also fibroblast growth, regulates the hepatic acute phase glycoprotein synthesis and is a principal mediator of fever in mammalian species (endogenous pyrogen) (reviewed in reference 29). Most relevant to the investigations of IL-1 CSF are the demonstration of IL-1 (1) to induce prostaglandin synthesis when applied on cortical slices,[30] (2) to cause a febrile response and an increase of slow wave sleep (SWS) activity when injected intracerebro-ventricularly,[31,32] (3) to influence neuro-endoctrine pathways by, for example, reducing opioid binding[33] or inducing corticotropin releasing factor secretion,[34] and (4) to induce an increase in astrocyte growth.[35] The receptor for IL-1α has been shown to be identical to that for IL-1β on both murine and human cells. Brain sections incubated with [^{125}I]-IL-1 also demonstrated a distinctive pattern of IL-1 receptor distribution mostly on neuronal cells that was widespread throughout the brain.[36] Additionally, affinity crosslinking studies indicate that the rat brain IL-1 receptor shares similarities with the IL-1 binding sites described on T cells and fibroblasts.[36] An IL-1 like activity has been demonstrated in supernatants of cultured astrocytes[37] as well as in extracts of brain from either mice being injected intraperitoneally with endotoxin[38] or from rats with brain lesions.[39] A few studies have focused on IL-1 in CSF samples.

In a thorough study on CSF from patients with noninflammatory neurologic diseases (eg, disc herniation, cervical spondylosis, spondylolisthesis and degenerative disc disease) IL-1 was detected when using the mitogen costimulation assay with mouse thymocytes or the IL-1 dependent IL-2 secretion by LBRM-1A5B6 cells. Upon fractionation on G-100 columns most of the activity eluted in fractions with corresponding molecular weights of 15 kDa and 30 kDa.[40] This is in contrast to a recent study showing no IL-1 like activity in CSF of control subjects undergoing myelograms. However, patients with severe head injury had detectable ventricular fluid IL-1 activities as shown by testing Sephadex G-50 fractions of ventricular fluids in the thymocyte assay.[41] In strain 13 guinea pigs with chronic relapsing experimental allergic encephalitis due to immunization with homologous spinal cord in complete Freund's adjuvant, Il-1 was detected in the thymocyte assay in CSF of animals with postacute, relapse or remission phases of disease.[42] On sephacryl S-200 the IL-1 peak appeared in fractions with an apparent molecular weight of 15 kDa.

In experiments with systemically administered IL-1 or endotoxin no IL-1 was detected in the CSF of the experimental animals, indicating impermeability of the blood brain barrier for IL-1.[43] This is in contrast to the studies with systemic IL-2 infusions which were followed by the appearance of IL-2 in lumbar CSF 4-6 hr later.[44] The CSF pharmacokinetics contrasted with the rapid elimination of IL-2 from plasma and demonstrated significant blood-CSF barrier penetration.[44]

Taken together, there is evidence for an IL-1 like activity in CSF or ventricular fluids of some patients or even non-inflammatory controls when tested in the thymocyte assay. However, at least one other cytokine, BSF-2, has been found to have effects on thymocytes which are not distinguishable from those observed with IL-1.[45] Therefore, future studies have to be carried out by taking the advantage of the availability of antibodies against IL-1α, IL-1β and BSF-2/IL-6.

CONCLUSION

The analysis of CSF for the presence of cytokines offers a strategy which in general will help to define the role of cytokines in inflammatory reactions *in-vivo.* More specifically, the demonstration of intrathecal synthesis of cytokines will contribute to the question on possible participation of brain parenchymal cells in the regulation of immune processes taking place in the CNS. For instance, the detection of intrathecal production of BSF-2 in viral infections of the CNS, together with the *in vitro* finding of synthesis of BSF-2 by virus-infected astrocytes and microglial cells, strongly favors the hypothesis that the intrathecal synthesis of antiviral immunoglobulins by B cells infiltrating the brain parenchyma is supported by glial cells in the brain. Furthermore, high levels of IFNγ in the CSF in T cell mediated viral diseases may induce the expression of MHC class I and II antigens on brain parenchymal cells and meningeal cells; this will enable facultative antigen presenter cells (APC) to fulfill their function and to present antigens to T/B cells invading the CNS. TNFα produced intrathecally in bacterial meningitis may be the key mediator for the initiation of the meningal inflammatory response. In further studies the regulation of cytokine production in the CNS has to be addressed.

REFERENCES

1. A. Fontana, K. Frei, S. Bodmer, and E. Hofer, Immune-mediated encephalitis: on the role of antigen-presenting cells in brain tissue, *Immunol.Rev.*, 100:185-201 (1987).
2. K. Frei, T.P. Leist, A. Meager, P. Gallo, D. Leppert, R.M. Zinkernagel, and A. Fontana, Production of B cell stimulatory factor-2 and interferon in the central nervous system during viral meningitis and encephalitis. Evaluation in a murine model infection and in patients, *J.Exp.Med.*, 168:449-453 (1988).
3. P. Lebon, B. Boutin, O. Dulac, G. Ponsot, and M. Arthuis, Interferon γ in acute and subacute encephalitis, *Br.Med.J.*, 296:9-11 (1988).
4. R. L. Hirsh, H.S. Panitch, and K.P. Johnson, Lymphocytes from multiple sclerosis patients produce elevated levels of gamma interferon in vitro, *J.Clin.Immunol.*, 5:386-389 (1985).
5. P. Lebon, E. Schuller, J.-D. Degos, O. Lyon-Caen, and G. Ponsot, CSF alpha and gamma interferons in acute and subacute encephalitis and multiple sclerosis: comparative study, in: 'Cellular and Humoral Immunological Components of Cerebrospinal Fluid in Multiple Sclerosis,' A. Lowenthal, J. Raus, eds., Plenum Publishing Corporation, pp. 429-436 (1987).

6. T. R. Moench and D.E. Griffin, Immunocytochemical identification and quantitation of the mononuclear cells in the cerebrospinal fluid, meninges, and brain during acute viral meningoecephalitis, *J.Exp.Med.*, 159:77-82, (1984).
7. U. Traugott, E. Shevach, J. Chiba, S.H. Stone, and C.S. Raine, Acute experimental autoimmune encephalomyelitis: T- and B-cell distribution within the target organ, *Cell Immunol.*, 70:345-356 (1982).
8. W. W. Tourtellotte, and B.I. Ma, Multiple sclerosis - the blood-brain-barrier and the measurement of de novo central nervous system IgG synthesis, *Neurology*, 28:76-83 (1978).
9. B. Vandvik, and E. Norrby, Oligoclonal IgG antibody response in the central nervous system to different measles virus antigens in subacute sclerosing panecephalitis, *Proc.Natl.Acad.Sci.*USA, 70: 1060-1063 (1973).
10. H. Link, Cerebrospinal fluid in immunological CNS diseases, *in:* 'Clinical Neuroimmunology,' J.A. Aarli, W.M.H. Behan and P.O. Behan, eds., Blackwell Scientific Publications, Oxford, pp. 444-466 (1987).
11. T. J. Kishimoto, B-cell stimulatory factors: molecular structure, biological function, and regulation of expression, *Clin.Immunol.*, 7:343-355 (1987).
12. J. Van Snick, S. Cayphas, A. Vink, C. Uyttenhove, P.G. Coulie, M.R. Rubira and R.J. Simpson, Purification and NH2-terminal amino acid sequence of a T-cell-derived lymphokine with growth factor activity for B-cell hybridomas, *Proc.Natl.Acad.Sci.*USA, 83:9679-9683 (1986).
13. J. Content, L. De Wit, P. Poupart, G. Opdenakker, J. Van Damme, and A. Billiau, Induction of a 26 kDa protein mRNA in human cells treated with an interleukin-l-related, leukocyte derived factor, *Eur.J.Biochem.*, 152:253-257 (1985).
14. A. Zilberstem, R. Ruggieri, J.H. Korn, and M. Revel, Structure and expression of cDNA and genes for human interferon 2, a distinct species inducible by growth-stimulatory cytokines, *EMBO J.*, 5:2529-2537, (1986).
15. H. Kikutani, T. Taga, S. Akira, H. Kishi, Y. Miki, O. Saiki, Y. Yamamura, and T. Kishimoto, Effects of B cell differentiation factor on biosynthesis and secretion of immunoglobulin molecules in human B cell lines, *J.Immunol.*, 134:990-995 (1985).
16. A. Muraguchi, T. Hirano, B. Tang, T. Matsuda, Y. Horii, K. Nakajima, and T. Kishimoto, The essential role of B cell stimulatory factor 2 for the terminal differentiation of B cells, *J.Exp.Med.*, 167:332-244 (1988).
17. R. Ceredig, J.E. Allan, Z. Tabi, F. Lynch, and P.C. Doherty, Phenotypic analysis of the inflammatory exudate in murine lymphocytic choriomeningitis, *J.Exp.Med.*, 165:1539-1551 (1987).
18. J. Baenziger, H. hengartner, R.M. Zinkernagel, and G.A. Cole, Induction or prevention of immunopathological disease by cloned cytotoxic T cell lines specific for lymphocytic choriomeningitis virus, *Eur.J.Immunol.*, 16:387-392 (1986).
19. A. Fontana, K. Frei, U.V. Malipiero, T.P. Leist, R.M. Zinkernagel, and M.E. Schwab, On the cellular source and function of B cell stimulatory factor 2/interleukin 6 produced in the central nervous system in viral diseases, (submitted).
20. P. B. Sehgal, D.C. Helfgott, U. Santhanam, S.B. Tatter, R.H. Clarick, J.Ghrayed, and L.T. May, Regulations of the acute phase and immune responses in viral disease. Enhanced expression of the 2-interferon/hepatocyte-stimulating factor/interleukin-6 gene in virus infected human fibroblasts, *J.Exp.Med.*, 167:1051-1956 (1988).
21. F. A. Houssiau, K. Bukasa, C.J.M. Sindic, J.Van Damme, and J.Van Snick, Elevated levels of the 26 K human hybridoma growth factor (interleukin-6) in cerebrospinal fluid of patients with acute infection of the central nervous system, *Clin.Exp.Immunol.*, 71:320-323 (1988).
22. L. J. Old, Tumor necrosis factor, *Scientific Am.*, 43-49 (1988).

23. B. Beutler, and A. Cerami Cachectin: more than a tumor necrosis factor, *N.Engl.J.Med.*, 316:379-385 (1987).
24. D. S. Robbins, Y. Shirazi, B.E., Drysdale, A. Lieberman, H.S. Shin, and M.L. Shin, Production of cytotoxic factor for oligodendrocytes by stimulated astrocytes, *J.Immunol.*, 139:2593-2597 (1987).
25. P. Scuderi, K.E. Sterling, K.S. Lam, P.R. Finley, K.J. Ryan, C.G. Ray, E. Petersen, D.J. Slymen and S.E. Salmon, Raised serum levels of tumor necrosis factor in parasitic infections, *Lancet*, 2:1364-1365 (1986).
26. A. Waage, A. Halstensen and T. Espevik, Association between tumor necrosis factor in serum and fatal outcome in patients with meningococcal disease, *Lancet* 1, 355-357 (1987).
27. E. P. Leist, K. Frei, S. Kam-Hansen, R. Zinkernagel, and A. Fontana, Tumor necrosis factor α in cerebrospinal fluid during bacterial, but not viral meningitis, *J.Exp.Med.*, 167:1743-1748 (1988).
28. P. Gallo, D. Kaegi, K. Frei, D. Leppert, D. Nadal, H. Lamche, C. Mueller, T. Leist, H. Hengartner, and A. Fontana, Production of tumor necrosis factor α in the central nervous system in infectious meningitis, (submitted).
29. C. A. Dinarello, An update oń human interleukin-1: from molecular biology to clinical relevance, *J.Clin.Immunol.*, 5:287-297 (1985).
30. C. A. Dinarello and H.A. Bernheim, Ability of human leukocytic pyrogen to stimulate brain prostaglandin synthesis in vitro, *J.Neurochem.*, 37:702-708 (1981).
31. J. M. Krueger, J. Walter, C.A. Dinarello, S.M. Wolff and L. Chedid, Sleep-promoting effects of endogenous pyrogen (interleukin-1), *Am.J.Physiol.*, 246:R994-R999 (1984).
32. I. Tobler, A.A. Borbély, M. Schwyzer, and A. Fontana, Interleukin-1 derived from astrocytes enhances slow wave activity in sleep EEG of rat, *Eur.J.Pharmacol.*, 104:191-192 (1984).
33. M. S. Ahmed, J. Leanos-Q, C.A. Cinarello and C.M. Blatteis, Interleukin-1 reduces opiod binding in guinea pig brain, *Peptides* 6, 1149-1154 (1985).
34. F. Berkenbozch, J. van Oers, A. del Rey, F. Tilders, and H. Besedovsky, Corticotropin-releasing factor-producing neurons in the rat activated by interleukin-1., *Science* 238:524-526 (1987).
35. D. Giulian and L.B. Lachman, Interleukin-1 stimulation of astroglial proliferation after brain injury, Science, 228:497-499 (1985).
36. W. L. Farrar, P.L. Kilian, M.R. Ruff, J.M. hill, and C.B. Pert, Visualization and characterization of interleukin-1 receptors in brain, *J.Immunol.*, 139:459-463 (1987).
37. A. Fontana, F. Kristensen, R. Dubs, D. Gemsa, and E. Weber, Production of prostaglandin E and an interleukin 1 like factor by cultured astrocytes and C-6 glioma cells, *J.Immunol.*, 129:2413-2419 (1982).
38. A. Fontana, E. Weber and J.M. Dayer, Synthesis of interleukin-1/endogenous pyrogen in the brain of endotoxin-treated mice: a step in fever induction? *J.Immunol.*, 133:1696-1698 (1984).
39. M. Nieto-Sampedro and M.A. Berman, Interleukin-1-like activity in rat brain: sources, targets, and effects of injury, *J.Neuroscience Res.*, 17:214-219 (1987).
40. R. M. Gorczynski, and E.J. Keystone, Interleukin-1-like activity in human cerebrospinal fluid, *Immunol.Lett.* 13., 231-235 (1986).
41. C. J. McClain, D. Cohen, L. Ott, C.A. Dinarello and B. Young, Ventricular fluid interleukin-1 activity in patients with head injury, *J.Lab.Clin.Med.*, 110:48-54 (1987).
42. J. A. Symons, R.V. Bundick, A.J. Suckling and M.G. Rumsby, Cerebrospinal fluid interleukin-1 like activity during chronic relapsing experimental allergic encephalomyelitis, *Clin.exp.Immunol.*, 68:648-654 (1987).
43. F. Coceani, J. Lees, and C.A. Dinarello, Occurrence of interleukin-1 in cerebrospinal fluid of the conscious cat, *Brain Res.*, 446:245-250 (1988).

44. S. C. Saris, S.A. Rosenberg, R.B. Friedman, J.T. Rubin, D. Barba and E.H. Oldfield, Penetration of recombinant interleukin-2 across the blood-cerebrospinal fluid barrier, *J.Neurosurg.*, 69:29-34 (1988).
45. C. Wyttenhove, P.G. Coulie, and J.T. van Snick, cell growth and differentiation induced by interleukin-HP1/IL-6, the murine hybridoma/plasmocytoma growth factor, *J.Exp.Med.*, 167:1417-1427 (1988).

IMMUNOCOMPETENT-LIKE CELLS IN HUMAN FETAL BRAIN CULTURES

M.G. Ennas, S. Torelli, V. Sogos, C. Marcello*, A. Riva and F. Gremo

Department of Cytomorphology and
*Institut of Obstetrics and Gynecology, School of Medicine, Cagliari, Italy

INTRODUCTION

The role played by endogenous brain cells in the pathogenesis of several diseases of the human Central Nervous System (CNS) is still rather obscure. In brain, besides neurons, other cells are present, like microglial cells, which are believed to be macrophage precursors and have been shown to express *in vitro* Fc receptors and to phagocytose.[1] Moreover, the presence of pluripotential hemopoietic stem cells in adult mouse brain has been reported.[2] Recent studies have also shown that astrocytes can act as macrophages[3] and, under appropriate stimulation, as antigen-presenting cells.[4] Purified astrocyte cultures from mammalian brain can produce interleukin I, II and III-like molecules, [5,6] further substantiating the hypothesis that glial cells can play an autonomous role in the immunological events of CNS.

In humans, very little information is available. However, in the last few years, data have been collected which show that cultured glial cells from human brain can express antigens of the major histocompatibility complex-class II either spontaneously[7,8] or under exogenous stimulation.[9,10] In previous work, we have developed and characterized cultures from human fetal brain of different stages of gestation.[11] In this report, we present the results about the spontaneous expression of several antigens which are markers for different classes of immunocompetent cells (macrophages, B and T lymphocytes), by human brain cells in culture.

MATERIALS AND METHODS

Preparation of Tissue Cultures

Human brains, obtained from either spontaneous or medically induced abortions, were freshly dissected and, when possible, divided into regions. Tissues were incubated with 0.2% sterile trypsin and dissociated into single cells by flushing through a Pasteur pipette. The cell suspension was diluted to 2×10^6 cells/ml in DMEM (Dulbecco's Modified Eagle Medium) plus 10% FCS (fetal calf serum). Cells were plated on plastic culture dishes pretreated with polylysine (PL). PL-dishes were prepared according to Pettmann et al.[12]

Immunocytochemistry

Glass coverslips (12 mm in diameter) were dropped into the plastic dish before PL treatment. At different times, coverslips were removed from dishes and routinely fixed at -20°C with cold methanol for 4 min. Samples were kept at -20°C until staining.

For the staining, samples were washed with Tris-HCl buffer (0.05 M, pH 7.4) plus Triton X-100 (0.4%). The excess of liquid was dried out and samples were covered with 20 µl of antibody solution (2 mg/ml final concentration in buffer). For characterization of cultures, monoclonal antibodies used were against: glial fibrillary acidic protein (GFA-P), vimentin (VT), desmin (DM), the major subunits of neurofilaments (NF 68K, 160K and 200K), all from Boeringher and against A2B5 (from Seralab); polyclonal antibodies against galactocerebroside (GalCb) from Chemicon. Also, fluorescent peanut lectin (PNA) from Sigma was used. The other antibodies used for immunocytochemistry are summarized in Table 1. After incubation at room temperature for 30 min, samples were washed three times with buffer. Then, they were incubated at room temperature for 30 min with 20 µl of fluorescent anti-mouse antibodies. For double staining, polyclonal antibodies against neurofilaments (a gift from Dr Dahl) or against glial fibrillary acidic protein (Dako) were used. In the latter case, after the two-step incubation with the monoclonal plus fluorescent anti-mouse antibodies, a second two-step incubation with polyclonal plus rhodamine-labeled anti-rabbit antibodies (1:20) was performed. After three washes, samples were dried and mounted. In order to test the effect of fixation on antigen preservation, some samples were incubated unfixed with either the first or with the first and the second antibody and then fixed with methanol as above. In both cases, Triton X-100 was omitted

Table 1. Panel of antibodies used for immunocytochemistry in fetal human brain cultures

Antibody	Antigen	Source	Specificity
OKB_2		Ortho	Mature and immature B lymph. membr.
OKB_7		Ortho	B lymph. membr.
HLA-DR		Ortho/Becton Dick.	B lymph ++/mon./macr.
OKT_4	CD4	Ortho/*Malavasi	T helper
OKT_8	CD8	Ortho/*Malavasi	T suppressor/cytotox.
OKT_9		Ortho	Trans. Recept.
OKT_{11}	CD2	Ortho	Pan T
Thy.1		Seralab	Immature thymocytes
OKNK		Ortho	Natural killer
LEU_7		Becton Dick.	Natural killer
A_{10}		*Malavasi	Activate lymph.
OKM_1	CD15	Ortho	Monocytes
OKM_5		Ortho	Monocytes, platelets
C_3bR	CD35	Dako	B lymph, pmn, macr.
S100		Ortho/Dako	Glia, melanocytes
Vimentin		Dako/Boeringher	Mesenchymal cells
Factor VIII		Dako	Endothelial cells
Fibronectin		*Tarone	Fibroblasts
IL2r (TAC)	CD25	Becton Dick./*Malavasi	
IL1	IL1	*Malavasi	

* Dr F. Malavasi and Dr G. Tarone, Department of Genetics, Biology and Biochemistry, School of Medicine, Torino, Italy.

from the buffer. In some cases preincubation with goat serum was used in order to block non-specific labeling. However, since no appreciable differences were detected, this passage was generally omitted.

Scanning Electron Microscope Immunocytochemical Staining

Cultured cells were prefixed in a solution containing 0.1% glutaraldehyde in 0.1 M cacodylate buffer plus 0.1% M sucrose for 15 min at 37°C and for additional 15 min at room temperature. After washes with PBS plus sucrose,, samples were incubated with the monoclonal antibody for 30 min. This step was followed by incubation with anti-mouse antibodies labeled with gold particles (size = 5 nm). Samples were then post-fixed with 2% glutaraldehyde in cacodylate buffer for 60 min at room temperature. After three washes in buffer and three more washes in distilled water, samples were incubated with solution for silver enhancement (kit by Janssen) for 9-18 min and then dehydrated with acetone and critical point dried using carbondioxide. Specimens were then briefly coated (1.5 min) with gold-palladium in a 5100 'cool' Polaron sputtering apparatus and observed with an ISI SS40 scanning electron microscope operating at 20 Kv.

RESULTS

Characterization of Human Brain Cultures

Specific markers were used to identify cell types in our cultures. As shown in Table 2, neurons were present in our cultures longer than two months. After three months, they died and only non-neuronal cells were present. Neurons very seldom grew isolated but generally formed clusters growing on the top of non-neuronal cells. A well developed network of processes was present already after two weeks in culture. Very often, the growing processes contacted and even wound around the cell bodies (Fig.1). Results also showed that no GalCb+ cells were present, not even at later stages of pregnancy, even if A2B5+ cells were always detectable. Thus, no oligodendrocytes developed, even if the common precursor to oligodendrocytes and type II astrocytes was indeed present.[13] On the contrary, the percentage of GFA-P+ cells, i.e. type II astrocytes, increased with time in culture, so that the older the age of the fetus, the earlier the expression of the protein. GFA-P+ cells showed a range of morphological features. At early stages, a few, round-shaped cells showing a more diffused staining for GFA-P were present. Later on, the cells became flatter with extending processes and had protein arranged in filaments (Fig. 2a and b). Very low (less than 2%) contamination from fibroblasts occurred in our cultures. Contamination by endothelial cells was excluded by the negativity of staining for factor VIII.

Table 2. Human fetal primary cultures: *in toto* brain

Age (weeks)	Days (in vitro)	NF160	NF200	GC	VT	FN	GFA-P	VIII	A2B5
7-8	10	-	+	-	+++	-	-	-	nd
12	17	+	+++	-	++	-	-	-	++
13	32	++	+++	-	++	±	++	-	nd
17	70	+	++	-	++	±	++	-	+

nd = Not determined.

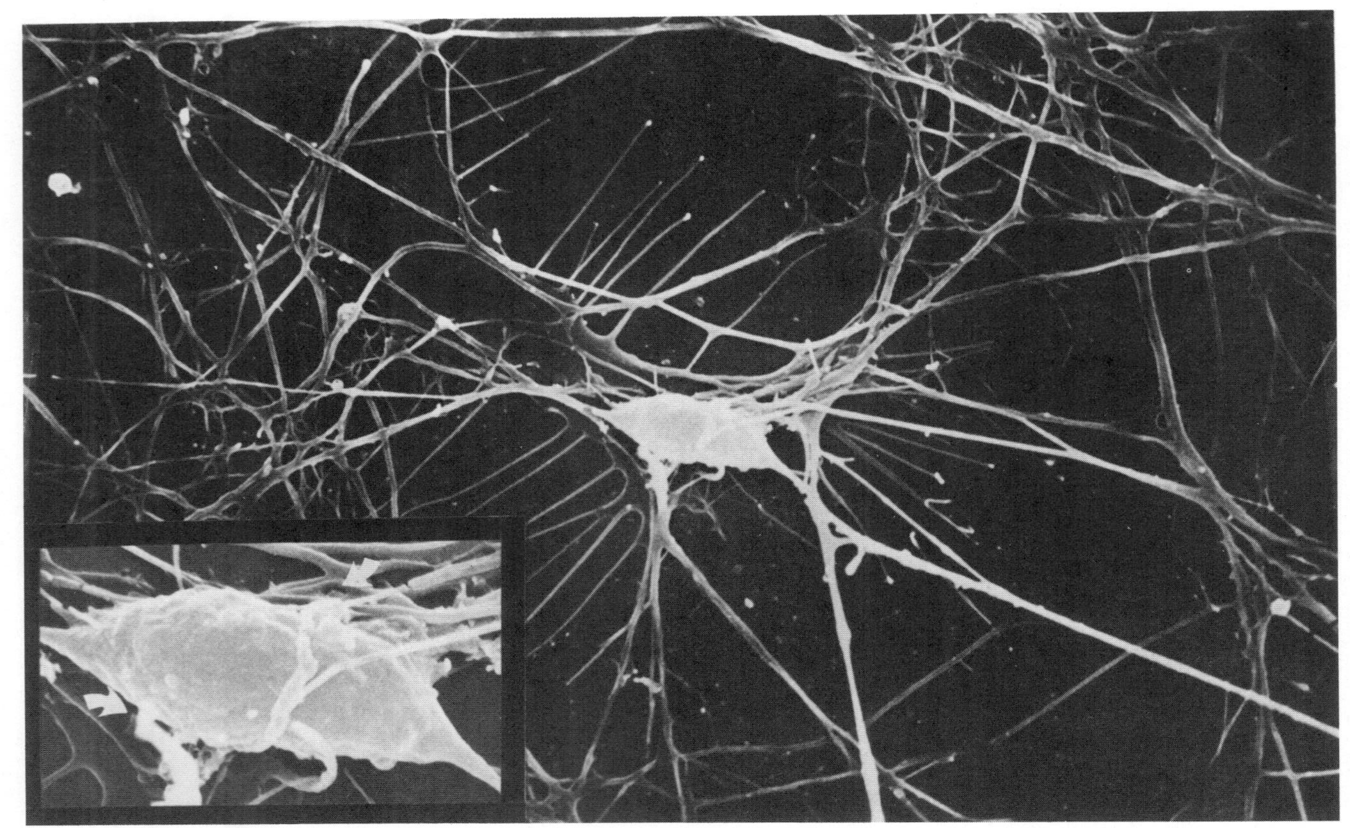

Fig. 1. Scanning electron microscopy (SEM) of human brain cultures (12-week-old embryo, Day 20 *in vitro*). Magnification of a neuron, with a well developed network of processes (X 8000). Square: Fibers contact the cell body and can even be wound around it (arrow). Magnification: X 18,500.

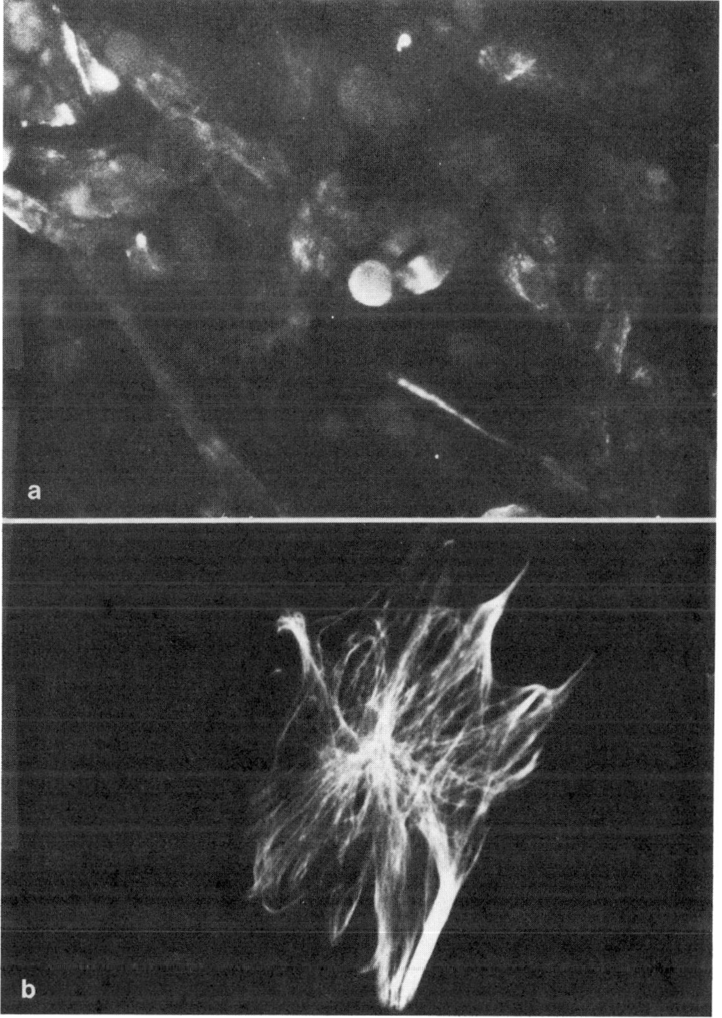

Fig. 2. GFA-P staining of human fetal brain cultures (12-week-old embryo). (a) Day 10 *in vitro*. Within the first two weeks in culture, very few cells express GFA-P, which is mostly present on the surface of round-shaped cells. A weak staining is detectable on flat cells. (b) Day 40 *in vitro*. With time in culture, most of the astrocytes become GFA-P positive; the protein is arranged in filaments. Magnification = X 400.

Localization of Immunocompetent Cell Antigens

Table 3 summarizes the results obtained with the panel of antibodies against the immunocompetent cell antigens. They show that type II astrocytes (GFAP+) bore all the antigens, with the exception of T9 and T11. T8 labeling was weak and could depend on the source of antibodies. On the contrary, neurons were positive only for B2 and CD4 (only a few). H-NK positive astrocytes were extremely rare, but Thy1, CD4 (Fig. 3) and A10 antigens were extremely diffused on astrocytes. Interestingly, among the macrophage typical markers, M1 was widely distributed (Fig. 4), whereas M5 staining was much less often observed. S-100 was most of the time negative. A weak staining was present only at the

Table 3. Localization of typical antigens of immunocompetent cells in cultured human brain cells

	Markers	Neurones	Astrocytes
B Lymphocytes			
	B2	+	+
	B7	-	++
	HLA-DR	-	++
T Lymphocytes			
	T4	- (+)	+
	T8	-	-
	T9	-	-
	T11	-	-
	Thy.1	+	+
	H-NK	-	-
	PNA	+	++
Macrophages			
	M1	-	+
	M5	-	+
	C3b	-	+
	S-100	-	-
	VT	+	+
	Fag.act.	-	-

latest stages of gestation and several weeks were necessary before the cells were able to express this glial protein. PNA receptor was present on both neurons and astrocytes. The staining was heavy and diffused. Very few round-shaped cells had the receptor for the Fc fragment of the antibodies.

DISCUSSION

Characterization of Human Cultures

The use of specific markers demonstrated that our cultures were enriched with neurons, astrocytes and their precursors and that there was no contamination by endothelial cells. Despite the fact that A2B5+ cells were indeed detectable, none of them developed into oligodendrocytes. This observation is in accord with Elder and Major,[14] who also reported the absence of oligodendrocytes in brain cultures of early human embryos. Since we extended the observations much further, these results parallel the phenomenon of late myelinization in the human species. Also Yong et al[15] reported the absence of oligodendrocytes in fetal brain cultures. On the contrary, Mauerhoff et al[10] found some oligodendrocytes in human brain cultures from 11-19 weeks of gestation. However, the cells were plated on glass and not on polylysine. Thus, the substratum we used might have contrasted the development of oligodendrocytes. In accord with the same author we also observed a rapid growth of astrocytes, which increased with fetal age and time in culture.

Localization of Antigens for Immunocompetent Cells

All the antigens we tested were present in brain cells, with the exception of T9 and T11. There is increasing evidence that many antigens which are present on immunocompetent cells can also be detectable in the brain. Antigens of a non-T, non-B acute-lymphocytic-leukemia cell line were detected also in human brain.[16] The structure of brain antigen proteins was reported to be very similar to that of leukemia cells, indicating that there was not cross-reactivity. On the contrary, HNK-1 (Leu7), a monoclonal antibody reactive with a subpopulation of human peripheral blood natural killer lymphocytes, has been reported to react

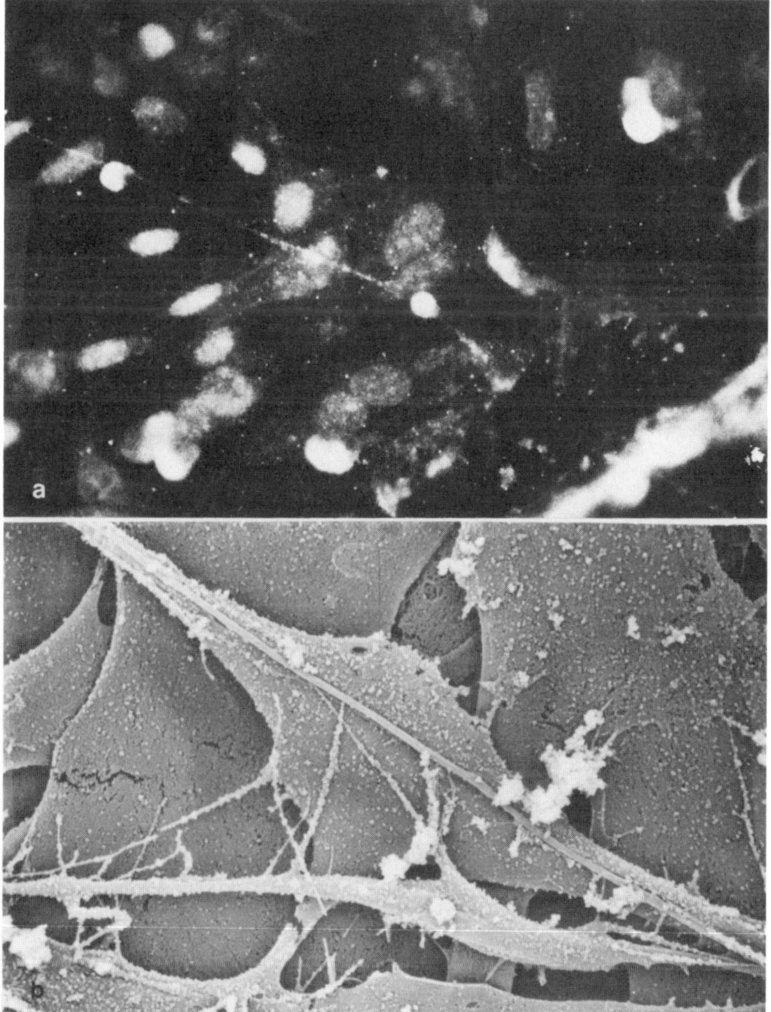

Fig. 3. M1 staining of human fetal brain cultures (12-week-old embryo). (a) Fluorescent staining shows that the antigen is widely diffused on astrocytes (identified with double staining with GFA-P antibody, not shown here). Magnification = X 500. (b) SEM staining shows that the antigen is present on the surface of cells with morphological features of astrocytes. Some processes are heavily stained, whereas others are completely negative (arrow). Magnification = X 17,400.

with the white matter of the central and peripheral nervous systems.[17,18] It has been shown to react with myelin-associated protein (MAG)[18] and with N-CAM, as well as neural adhesion molecules[19] which have a common epitope. Thus, the weak reactivity we observed in our cultures could be due to any of the above phenomena.

Thy1-like immunoreactivity is indeed present in human brain during development.[20] According to Granholm et al[20] the antigen was detectable in both white and grey matter. We found that both neurons and astrocytes expressed this antigen, as already shown in other mammals.[21]

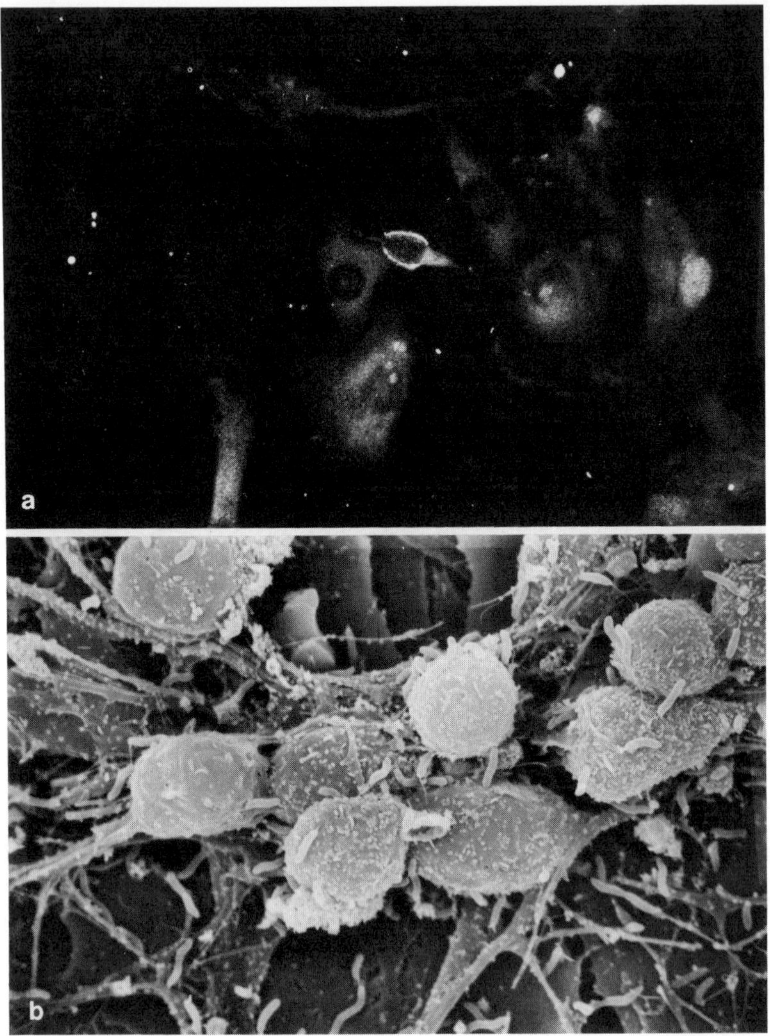

Fig. 4. Expression of CD4. (a) Immunofluorescent staining. Magnification = X 400. (b) SEM immunocytochemical staining. Magnification = X 11,000. This typical marker of T lymphocytes is expressed on the surface of cells with different morphology. Double staining (not shown here) indicate that some are astrocytes and a few are neurons.

It is of great interest that CD4 was inequivocably detectable on type II astrocytes. In fact, Maddon et al[22] have shown that CD4 antigen is indeed present in human brain, but they were unable to identify the type of cell expressing this antigen. To our knowledge, this is the first demonstration that this antigen is expressed by human fetal astrocytes from very early stages of development. It could explain the susceptibility of nervous tissue to infection by immunodeficiency virus, which is indeed restricted to the cells which express T4 glycoprotein on their surface.[23,24] Unknown, is the role of CD4 during brain development. However, we have demonstrated that HLA-DR antigen is present in brain cells.[8] The hypothesis can be advanced that interaction between CD4 and class II antigens could be involved in cell recognition during the formation of neuronal pattern in brain development, as it has been hypothized for Thy1.[20]

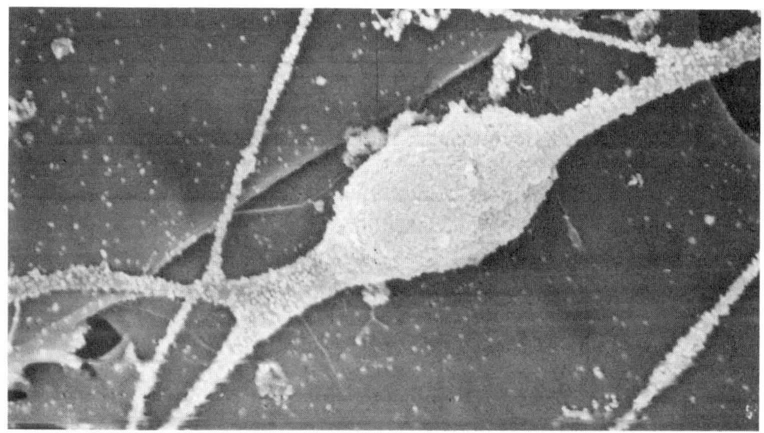

Fig. 5. B_2 expression on neuronal cells. The antigen is particularly abundant on neurons. This neuron is completely coated with reaction products. Glial cells (underneath) are much less positive. Magnification = X 16,500

Also of great interest is the finding that our cells express TAC receptor and that its expression is enhanced by serum withdrawal. Since in our cultures interleukin I- II- and III-like molecules have been detected,[25] it can be speculated that they have control on cell proliferation also in the developing human brain, as already shown in other mammals.[26]

ACKNOWLEDGMENTS

This research was supported by MPI (40-60%) and Regione Autonoma Sardegna (Assessorato all'Igiene e Sanità).

REFERENCES

1. M. C. Raff, K.L. Fields, S.I. Hakomori, R. Mirsky, R.M. Pruss and J. Winter, Cell-type specific markers for distinguishing and studying neurones and the major classes of glial cells in culture, *Brain Res.*, 174:283-308 (1979).
2. P. F. Bartlett, Pluripotential hemopoietic stem cells in adult mouse brain, *Proc.Natl.Acad.Sci.* USA, 79:2722-2725 (1982).
3. H. Kusaka, A. Hirano, M.B. Bornstein, G.R.W. Moore, and C.S. Raine, Transformation of cells of astrocyte lineage into macrophage-like cells in organotypic cultures of mouse spinal cord, *J.Neural.Sci.*, 72:77-89 (1986).
4. A. Fontana, W. Fierz and H. Wekerle, Astrocytes present myelin basic protein to encephalitogenic T-cell lines, *Nature*, 307:273 (1984).
5. A. Fontana, F. Kristensen, R. Dubs, D. Gemsa, and E. Weber, Production of prostaglandin E and interleukin I-like factors by cultured astrocytes and C-6 glioma cells, *J.Immunol.*, 129:2413-2419 (1982).
6. K. Frei, S. Booder, C. Schwerdel, and A. Fontana, Astrocytes of the brain synthesize interleukin III-like factors, *J.Immunol.*, 135:4044-4047 (1985).
7. S. U. Kim, G. Moretto, and D.H. Shin, Expression of Ia antigens of the surface of human oligodendrocytes and astrocytes in culture, *J.Neuroimmunol*, 10:141-149 (1985).
8. M. G. Marrosu, M.G. Ennas, S. Torelli, V. Sogos, P. Puligheddu, U. Lecca, and F. Gremo, Spontaneous expression of Ia antigen (HLA-DR) in

cultured cells of human fetal brain at different stages of gestation this volume pages 103-109.

9. M. Pulver, S. Carrel, J.P. Mach, and N. De Tribolet, Cultured human fetal astrocytes can be induced by interferon-gamma to express HLA-DR, *J.Neuroimmunol.*, 14:123-133 (1987).

10. T. Mauerhoff, R. Pujol-Borrel, R. Mirakian, and G.F. Bottazzo, Differential expression and regulation of major histocompatibility complex (MHC) products in nueronal and glial cells of the human fetal brain, *J.Neuroimmunol.*, 18:271-289 (1988).

11. F. Gremo, S. Torelli, V. Sogos, A. Riva, C. Marcello, U. Lecca, Morphological and immunocitochemical characterization of human fetal brain cultures, *Soc.Neurosci.Abstract*, vol 13, part. II, p. 1119 (1987).

12. B. Pettmann, J.C. Louis, M. Sensenbrenner, Morphological and biochemical maturation of neurons cultured in the absence of glial cells, *Nature*, 281:378-380 (1979).

13. M. C. Raff, R.H. Miller, M. Noble, A glial progenitor cell that develops *in vitro* into a astrocyte of an oligodendrocyte depending on culture medium, *Nature*, 303:390-396 (1983).

14. G. A. Elder and E.O. Major, Early appearance of type II astrocytes in developing human fetal brain, *Dev.Brain Research*, 42:146-150 (1988).

15. V. W. Yong, S.U. Kim, and D.E. Pleasure, Growth factors for fetal and adult human astrocytes in culture, *Brain Res.*, 444:59-66 (1988).

16. E. J. Quackenbush, T.F. Cruz, M.A. Moscarello, and M. Le Tarte, Identification of three antigens in human brain associated with similar antigens of human leukaemic cells, *Biochem.J.*, 225:291-299 (1985).

17. S. Schuller-Petrovic, W. Gebhart, H.Lassmann, H.Rumpold, and D. Kraft, A shared antigenic determinant between natural killer cells and nervous tissue, *Nature* 306:179-181 (1983).

18. R. C. McGarry, S.L. Helfand, R.A. Quarles, and J.C. Roder, Recognition of myelin-associated glycoprotein by the monoclonal antibody HNK-I, *Nature*, 306:376-378, (1983).

19. J. Kruse, R. Mailhammer, H. Wernecke, A. Faissner, I. Sommer, C. Goridis, and M. Schachner, Neural cell adhesion molecules and myelin-associated glycoprotein share a common carbohydrate moiety recognized by monoclonal antibodies L2 and HNK-I., *Nature*, 311:153-155 (1984).

20. A. C. H. Granholm, P. Almquist, Å. Seiger, and L. Olson, Thy. 1-like immunoreactivity in human brain during development, *Brain Res.Bull.*, 17:107-212, (1986).

21. R. Mirsky and E.J. Thompson, Thy.1 (Theta) antigen on the surface of morphologically distinct brain cell types, *Cell* 4:95-101 (1975).

22. P. J. Maddon, A.G. Dalgleish, J.S. McDougal, P.R. Clapham, R.A. Weiss, and R. Axel, The T4 gene encodes the AIDS virus receptor and is expressed in the Immune System and the Brain, *Cell* 47:333-348 (1986).

23. A. G. Dalgleish, P.C.L. Beverley, P.R. Clapham, D.H. Crawford, M.F. Greaves, and R.A. Weiss, The CD4 (T4) antigen is an essential component of the receptor for the AIDS retrovirus, *Nature*, 312:763-766 (1984).

24. J. S. McDougal, A. Mawle, S.P. Cort, J.K.A. Micholson, G.D. Cross, J.A. Sheppler-Campbell, D. Hicks, and J. Sligh, Cellular tropism of the human retrovirus HTLV-III/LAV I. Role of T cell activation and expression of the T4 antigen, *J.Immunol.*, 135:3151-3162 (1985).

25. L. Lauro, Role of astroglia in CNS immune response, *Proc.Int.Symp., Trends in Neuroimmunology*, p. 34 (1988).

26. R. P Saneto, F. Chiappelli, and J.De Vellis, Interleukin-2 inhibition of oligodendrocyte progenitor cell proliferation depends on expression of the TAC receptor, *J.Neurosci.Res.*, 18:147-154 (1987).

ROLE OF ASTROGLIAL CELLS IN EXPERIMENTAL ALLERGIC ENCEPHALOMYELITIS

L. Massacesi, A. L. Abbamondi*, F. Sarlo,
E. Castigli, J. Olivotto, M. Vergelli and L. Amaducci

Department of Neurology, University of Florence
V. le Morgagni 85, 50134 Florence, and
*Institute of Neurology, Catholic University
Rome, Italy

ROLE OF FIBROUS GLIOSIS IN INFLAMMATORY LESIONS OF THE CENTRAL NERVOUS SYSTEM (CNS)

Introduction

Astrocyte reaction is among the prominent events occurring in CNS inflammatory lesions. Such reaction leads to a particular way of scarring resulting in fibrous gliosis. Reactive astrocytes show cell body and nucleus morphology larger than the two major types of astrocytes described in normal nervous tissue.[1,2] Reactive astrocytes also contain larger amounts of DNA,[3] intermediate filaments,[4] glial fibrillary acidic protein (GFAP)[5,6] and oxidoreductive enzyme activity.[7] These cells probably contribute also to the removal and phagocytosis of degenerating myelin.[4] *In vivo* reactive astrocytes probably originate from normal astrocytes undergoing hyperplasia and hypertrophy.[1,7-11] However, the inducing signals and the time course of this activation are still unknown.

In CNS inflammatory lesions oligodendrocytes maintain regenerative activity, as shown by the presence of axons with disproportionately thin myelin sheats at the edge of many chronic lesions.[12,13] In these areas, which are interpreted as remyelination areas, oligodendroglial hyperplasia is not uncommon, and a broad band of proliferating oligodendroglia has been observed for a distance into demyelinating lesions.[14]

On the other hand, even in totally demyelinated lesions, the axons are usually spared, and are maintained naked in a matrix of dense fibrous astrogliosis lacking in oligodendroglia.[14] In older lesions, however, axons may be reduced in number.

The expansion of fibrous astrogliosis, producing an unattractive environment for repair and for oligodendrocyte proliferation, largely accounts for the failure of remyelination occurring in the larger and older lesions.[14] Thus, the restriction of CNS inflammatory damage resulting from the control of astroglial reaction may usefully support the new therapeutical strategies, such as cell transplants or regeneration inducing molecules. As a consequence, it is of primary importance to deepen the mechanisms of astroglial cell activation and proliferation *in vivo*.

The aim of our study is to contribute to an understanding of the time course in astroglial cell activation and proliferation during inflammatory diseases of the CNS.

Since pathological studies in humans can provide only limited information on the early phases of CNS inflammatory lesion development, we studied astroglial cell activation in experimental autoimmune encephalomyelitis (EAE), an animal model of CNS inflammatory disease.

Time Course of Astroglial Cell Activation and Proliferation During EAE

EAE was induced in 6-8-week-old female Lewis rats by inoculation of lyophilized myelin in complete Freund's adjuvant. In these experimental conditions, we observed inflammatory cell infiltrates in the CNS beginning from Day 11 after immunization (ai). At the same day, spinal cord biochemical assays showed increased levels of two lysosomal enzyme activities (acid protease and beta-glucuronidase) and total DNA concentration (parametric measure of cellular infiltrates). Histochemical examination of the same spinal cords showed an increased staining for acid phosphatase, which is considered a marker for lysosomal activity. Such increase was observed both inside and at a distance from the perivascular infiltrates. Cells which showed increased staining inside the infiltrates were inflammatory cells, while those on the outside had the typical astrocyte nucleus and cell body morphology. This observation strongly suggests that endogenous nervous cells could contribute to the reported increase in lysosomal enzyme activity.[15]

Astrocytes undergo activation and proliferation in response to interleukin-1 (IL-1), a lymphomonokine released during the CNS inflammatory response.[16] Such an increase is therefore expectable in an inflammatory disease as EAE. We counted astrocytes in the spinal cord of immunized rats and compared their number to that of GFAP-positive cells (GFAP+). The increase rate of GFAP+ cells was similar to that of the cells identified as astrocytes by morphological criteria. A very early increase of these cells was observed from Day 12 ai, corresponding in time to the reported total DNA content increase in the same spinal cords (Figure 1).

This data suggests that the cells showing an increase in acid phosphatase activity at the onset of EAE, and identified as astrocytes with morphological criteria, were indeed astrocytes.

Taken together, the reported observations suggest that, in CNS inflammatory diseases, astrocytes proliferate and are activated earlier than expected during the first inflammatory cell infiltration.[17] This is probably a consequence of IL-release and edema, which are typical features of cell-mediated immune response within tissues. The remarkable and early hypertrophy of the lysosomal apparatus, observed in cells morphologically identified as astrocytes, suggests that the reported lysosomal enzyme activities may be considered as a marker of astrocyte activation.

EXPRESSION OF Ia ANTIGENS IN CNS DURING EAE

Introduction

It is well-known that the expression of class II major histocompatibiity complex (MHC) antigens (Ia) plays an important role in time and space expansion of the immune response during autoimmune diseases such as EAE.[18] Class II MHC antigens are constitutively expressed on certain cell types (B lymphocytes, monocytes, dendritic cells). In normal rat CNS, only occasional Ia positive (Ia+) cells were normally observed in the meninges, especially around blood vessels,[19] and none of them were observed in the parenchyma. On the other hand, Ia+

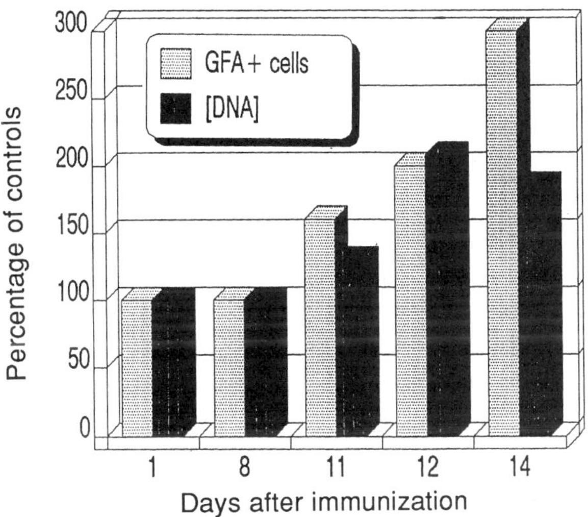

Fig. 1. Astrocytes and [DNA] increase in EAE: immunohistochemical and biochemical study.

cells are commonly observed in brain tissue during some immunomediated diseases. Traugott et al. for example observed Ia expression on endothelial cells and astrocytes in brain lesions during multiple sclerosis and mouse EAE.[20,21] Using double staining techniques, Hoffman et al. observed that most Ia+ cells were also GFAP+.[22] Similar data were reported by Sobel et al. in the guinea pig.[23-25] Furthermore, in SJL mice with acute or chronic-relapsing EAE induced by MBP-specific T-cell lines, parenchimal Ia+ cells were identified on serial sections as astrocytes.[26] Astrocytes have been reported to express Ia antigens *in vitro*: brain cell populations, consisting of approximately 90% astrocytes, have been cultured for 6-7 days and exposed to cloned gamma-interferon (γ-INF) for 24 hours. Only 15-20% of the total γ–INF-treated astrocytes expressed detectable Ia antigens in a double staining (Ia and GFAP), but this failure might be due either to the slow metabolic recovery of Ia-inducible cells or to the extremely low number of Ia-inducible cells in the initial cultures.[27]

Astrocytes have also been reported to act *in vitro* as antigen presenting cells (APC): γ-INF exposed Lewis rate astrocytes were co-cultured with myelin basic protein (MBP) and syngeneic MBP-specific T-cells. In these experimental conditions, astrocytes were able to carry out antigen presentation in a MHC-restricted manner.[28,29] Also CNS endothelial cells (EC) have been reported to act *in vitro* as APC: pretreatment of isolated murine CNS EC with concanavalin A conditioned media (ConA CM) resulted in Ia antigen expression; consequently, these cells were able to carry out antigen presentation to guinea pig MBP-sensitized murine lymphonode cell cultures.[30] The same *in vitro* activities were also shown by CNS EC freshly isolated from mice with adoptively transferred acute EAE.[31]

The reported *in vivo* and *in vitro* observations suggest that astrocytes and/or EC are the *in vivo* APC of the CNS. However, in Lewis rats with EAE, Matsumoto et al failed to detect Ia+ astrocytes.[32] The same results, in addition to failure of Ia+ EC detection, were obtained by Vass et al.[33] These observations revealed an important variability of results in different animal species and indicate that astrocytes and EC can act as APC in certain experimental conditions but not in others.

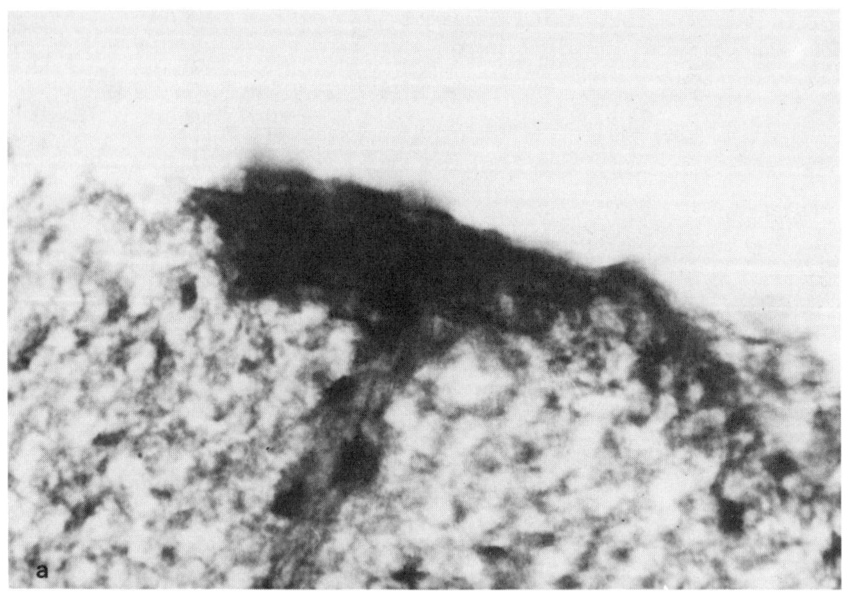

Fig. 2(a) Spinal cord of sensitized rat (Day 10). Mab OX6 + ABC; counterstained with haematoxylin. x 400. Ia+ cells are observed in the meninges and in the vessels near the surface of the spinal cord.

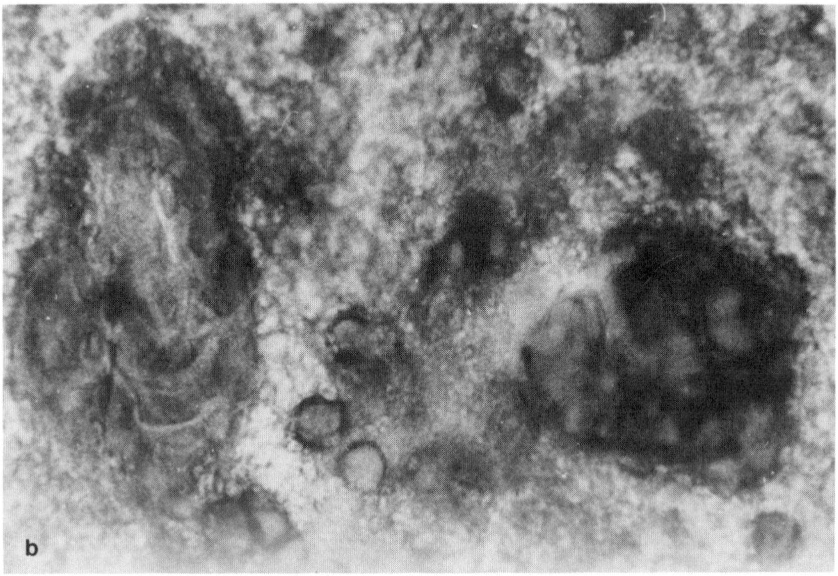

Fig. 2(b). Spinal cord of sensitized rat (Day 12). Mab OX6 + ABC; counterstained with haematoxylin x 1000. Many Ia+ cells are observed in the wall of the vessels and in the perivascular infiltrates.

Time Course of Ia Expression in CNS During EAE

We previously described in this report an early activation and proliferation of astrocytes during acute EAE. In order to correlate this data with the possible role of astrocytes in triggering or expanding the immune response during acute EAE, we tried to observe whether astrocytes could express Ia antigens at the onset of Lewis rat EAE and eventually act as APC *in vivo*.

A single staining technique was performed, using anti-rat Ia antigen monoclonal antibodies (Mabs) (Ox3-Ox6 SEROTEC) and the avidin-biotin technique. We also used a double staining with anti-Ia Mabs combined with anti-GFAP polyclonal antiserum, followed by an immunofluorescence technique. Both methods were employed on cryostate spinal cord sections taken from rats sacrificed at different stages of the disease.

The main results showed that one day before the onset of EAE (Day 10 ai) only few cells in the subpial region expressed Ia antigens, mainly around the vessels (Figure 2a). These cells had the morphology of inflammatory cells (lymphocytes, macrophages). At this stage of the disease, no Ia+ cells were observed outside the areas surrounding subpial vessels.

At Days 11 and 12 ai, corresponding to the onset of the disease, numerous Ia+ cells were observed in the perivascular infiltrates and in the nervous tissue (Figure 2b). The Ia+ cells observed in the perivascular infiltrates had the morphology of inflammatory cells. Moreover, CNS parenchymal Ia+ cells were negative for GFAP at the double staining observation.

In summary: (1) a moderate Ia expression was evident in the subpial regions, mainly around blood vessels, before the clinical onset of EAE. (2) Ia antigen expression increases during the inflammatory events. (3) Double staining with anti-Ia Mabs combined with GFAP antiserum did not show Ia+-GFAP+ cells.

According to Matsumoto et al,[32] and Vass et al,[33] these data suggest that astrocytes might not play a key role in the earlier antigen presentation in CNS, at least in Lewis rat acute EAE. This would confirm further observations by Matsumoto et al.[32] which indicate that the cells acting as the *in vivo* APC in the CNS are probably microglial.

The reported early activation of astrocytes might be triggered aspecifically by the inflammatory response itself, as can be observed in a variety of CNS injuries.

REFERENCES

1. P. Del Rio-Hortega and W. Penfield, Bull. Johns Hopkins Hosp., 31:278-303 (1927).
2. J. B. Cavanagh, *J. Anat.*, 106:471-487 (1970).
3. L. W. Lapham and M. A. Johnstone, *J. Neuropathol. Exp. Neurol.*, 23: 419-430 (1964).
4. E. J. H. Nathaniel and D. R. Nathaniel, *Exp. Neurol.*, 54:60-76 (1977).
5. A. Bignami and D. Dahl, *Neuropathol. Appl. Neurobiol.*, 2:99-111 (1976).
6. L. A. Amaducci, K. I. Forno and L. F. Eng, *Neurosci. Lett.*, 21:27-32 (1981).
7. M. Ochmichen, *Pathol. Res. Pract.*, 168:344-373 (1980).
8. N. Latov, G. Nilaver and A. Zimmerman, *Dev. Biol.*, 72:381-384 (1979).
9. C. P. Barret, L. Guth, E. G. Donati and J. G. Krikorian, *Exp. Neurol.*, 73:365-377 (1981).
10. E. J. H. Nathaniel and D. R. Nathaniel, "Advances in Cellular Neurobiology", vol. 2, Academic Press, New York, pp 249-301 (1981).

11. M. Polak, W. Haymaker, J. E. Johnson and D'Amelio, "Histology and Histopathology of the Nervous System", Vol. 1, Charles C. Thomas Pub.., Springfield, Illinois, pp 363-480 (1982).
12. J. W. Prineas and R. G. Wright, *Lab. Invest.*, 38:409-421 (1978).
13. C. S. Raine, *Lab. Invest.*, 50:608-635 (1982).
14. C. S. Raine, in: "Myelin", P. Morrel, ed., Plenum Press Pub., New York, N.Y., USA, pp 259-310 (1984).
15. L. Massacesi, A. L. Abbamondi, L. Raimondi, C. Giorgi and L. Amaducci, *Neurochem. Res.*, vol. 13 (2):165-169 (1988).
16. D. Giulian and L. B. Lachman, *Science*, vol. 228:497-499 (1985).
17. L. F. Eng, M. E. Smith and B. Gerstl, *in:* "Dynamic Properties of Glial Cells, Cellular and Molecular Aspects", T. Grisar, G. Franck, L. Hertz, W. T. Norton, M. Sensenbrenner and D. Woodbury, eds., Pergamon Press, Oxford, England, pp 1-8 (1986).
18. G. F. Bottazzo et al., *Lancet*, 2:1115 (1983).
19. W. Fierz and A. Fontana, in: "Cellular Neurobiology: Astrocytes", S. Feodoroff and A. Vernadakis, eds., Academic Press, New York, N. Y., p 203 (1986).
20. U. Traugott, L. C. Scheinberger and C. S. Raine, *J. Neuroimmunol.*, 8:1-14 (1985).
21. U. Traugott, C. S. Raine and D. E. McFarlin, *Cell. Immunol.*, 91:240 (1985).
22. F. M. Hoffman, R. F. von Hanwehr, C. A. Dinarello, S. B. Mizel, D. Hinton and J. E. Merrill, *J. Immunol.*, 136:3279 (1986).
23. R. A. Sobel, B. W. Blanchette, A. K. Bhan and R. B. Colvin, *J. Immunol.*, 132 (5):2393-2401 (1984).
24. R. A. Sobel, B. W. Blanchette, A. K. Bhan and R. B. Colvin, *J. Immunol.*, 132 (5): 2402-2407 (1984).
25. R. A. Sobel and R. B. Colvin, *J. Immunol.*, 134 (4):2333-2337 (1985).
26. K. Sakai, T. Tabira, M. Endoh and L. Steinman, *Lab. Invest.*, 54:345-352 (1986).
27. G. H. W. Wong, P. F. Bartlett, I. Clark-Lewis, J. L. McKimm-Breschkin and Schrader, *J. Neuroimmunol.*, 7:255-278 (1985).
28. A. Fontana, W. Fiertz and H. Wekerle, *Nature*, 307:273-276 (1984).
29. W. Fiertz, B. Endler, K. Reske, H. Wekerle and A. Fontana, *J. Immunol.*, 134 (6):3785-3793 (1985).
30. R. M. McCarron, O. Kempski, M. Spatz and D. McFarlin, *J. Immunol.*, 134 (5):3100-3103 (1985).
31. R. M. McCarron, M. Spatz, O. Kempski, R. N. Hogan, L. Muehl and D. E. McFarlin, *J. Immunol.*, 137 (11):3428-3435)1986).
32. Y. Matsumoto, N. Hara, R. Tanaka and M. Fujiwara, *J. Immunol.*, 136:3668 (1986).
33. K. Vass, H. Lassmann, H. Wekerle and H. M. Wisniewski, *Acta Neuropathol.* (Berl.), 70:149 (1986).

SPONTANEOUS EXPRESSION OF Ia ANTIGEN (HLA-DR) IN CULTURED CELLS OF HUMAN FETAL BRAIN AT DIFFERENT STAGES OF GESTATION

M. G. Marrosu, M. G. Ennas*, S. Torelli*, V. Sogos*, P. Puligheddu†, U. Lecca† and F. Gremo*

*Department of Cytomorphology, Institute of Child Neuropsychiatry
†Institute of Obstetrics and Gynecology, School of Medicine, Cagliari, Italy

INTRODUCTION

Antigens of the major histocompatibility complex (MHC) class II are known to play a key role in cell-mediated immune response. In the Central Nervous System (CNS), either none or very low percentages of Ia-positive cells have been detected in mouse or man.[1-5]

However, treatment with gamma-interferon dramatically increased the expression of Ia antigen in cultured astrocytes[3,6,7] as well as oligodendrocytes and neurons.[6] The conclusion drawn by these authors was that brain cells did not spontaneously express MHC-class II antigens unless an exogenous stimulation was applied. Moreover, Pulver et al[7] reported that brain cell lines from a 20-week-old human fetus had spontaneous but variable expression of HLA-DR antigens which could be up-regulated by treatment with recombinant gamma-interferon. On the contrary, Kim et al[5] reported the spontaneous expression of HLA-DR in oligodendrocytes and astrocytes from adult brain. These results are substantiated by a recent report by Mauerhoff et al[8] who showed that type II astrocytes could spontaneously express Ia antigen, even if this phenomenon was greatly enhanced by gamma interferon.

In this study, we investigated the spontaneous expression of Ia antigen in brain cultures of human fetuses, at different stages of gestation, for two reasons. First, it is important to know the timing of appearance of Ia-bearing cells under normal conditions; second, the origin and type of cells which spontaneously express HLA-DR antigens need to be known at a time in which the blood-brain barrier and the immune system are far from being mature. The presence of multipotent blood stem cells has been reported in mouse brain.[9] Thus, the fetal human brain provide a very useful system to test whether or not cells of brain origin can actually express antigens generally present in immunocompetent cells.

In addition, brain cultures offer advantages in respect to whole brain sections: they allow a precise location of the antigen since cells can be identified unambiguously by morphology plus the use of established markers. The actual presence of the antigen on cell surface might be masked by cell-cell contacts, which can lead to an underestimation of Ia molecules. Moreover, the fixation procedures which are often necessary for tissue sections reduce or abolish the detectability of Ia antigen and HLA-DR on cells.[10]

MATERIALS AND METHODS

Preparation of Tissue Cultures

Human brains, obtained from either spontaneous or medically induced abortions, were freshly dissected and, when possible, divided into regions. Tissues were incubated with 0.2% sterile trypsin and dissociated into single cells by flushing through a Pasteur pipette. The cell suspension was diluted to 2 x 10^6 cells/ml in DMEM (Dulbecco's Modified Eagle Medium) plus 10% FCS (fetal calf serum). Cells were plated on plastic culture dishes pretreated with polylysine (PL). PL-dishes were prepared according to Pettmann et al.[11]

Immunocytochemistry

Glass coverslips (12mm in diameter) were dropped into the plastic dish before PL treatment. At different times, coverslips were removed from dishes and routinely fixed at -20°C with cold methanol for 4 min. Samples were kept at -20°C until staining.

For the staining, samples were washed with Tris-HCl buffer (0.05 M, pH 7.4) plus Triton X-100 (0.4%). The excess of liquid was dried out and samples were covered with 20 µl of antibody solution (2 mg/ml final concentration in buffer).

Monoclonal antibodies were used from different sources against human HLA-DR (Dako, Ortho, Becton-Dickinson, Biotest). After incubation at room temperature for 30 min, samples were washed three times with buffer. Then, they were incubated at room temperature for 30 min with 20 µl of fluorescent anti-mouse. For double staining, polyclonal antibodies against neurofilaments (a gift from Dr Dahl) or against glial fibrillary acidic protein (GFA-P) (Dako) were used. In the latter case, after the two-step incubation with the anti-HLA-DR plus fluorescent anti-mouse antibody, a second two-step incubation with polyclonal plus rhodamine-labeled anti-rabbit antibodies (1:20) was performed. After three washes, samples were dried and mounted. In order to test the effect of fixation on antigen preservation, some samples were incubated unfixed with either the first or with the first and the second antibody and then fixed with methanol as above. In both cases, Triton X-100 was omitted from the buffer. In some cases preincubation with goat serum was used in order to block non-specific labeling. However, since no appreciable differences were detected, this passage was generally omitted.

Table 1. Expression of HLA-DR in Cultured Cells of Human Brain at Different Stages of Gestation

Days in culture	8 w	11-12 w	13 w	15-17 w	18-19 w
8-10	±	1%	1-2%	nd	nd (1%)*
14-16	nd	10% (1-2%)*	10%	30-50%	5% (1-2%)*
20-30	20%	30%	20-30*	10% (1-2%)*	20-30%
40-60	20%	50%	80%	1-2%	nd

* = Frontal cortex; nd = not determined; w = weeks of gestation.

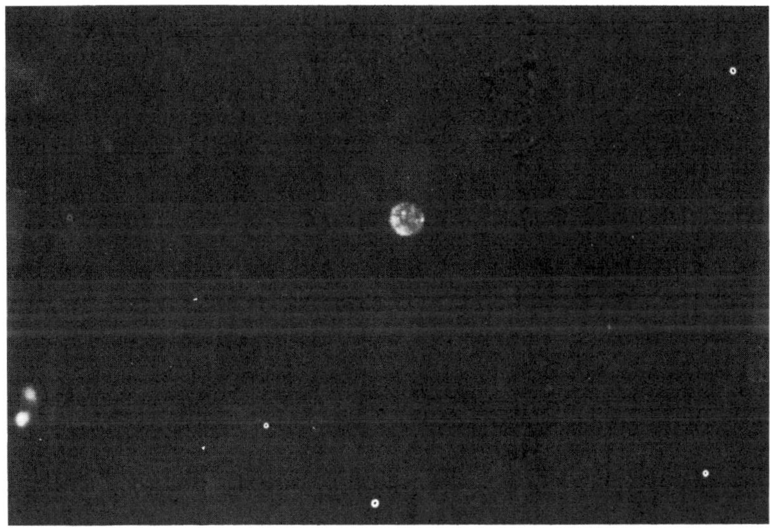

Fig. 1. HLA-DR expression on human fetal brain cells in culture (Day 8 *in vitro*). The antigen is distributed on cell surface of few round-shaped cells and absent on flat non neuronal cells. Magnification = X 400.

Immunocytochemistry at scanning electron microscopy (SEM) level was also performed. For details of the technique see Ennas et al.[12]

RESULTS

Results are summarized in Table 1. They show that in very early stages (8 weeks of pregnancy) there were indeed cells which spontaneously expressed HLA-DR after a few days in culture. This percentage was alike in all the stages considered. Later, the percentage of positive cells increased. It was significantly affected by fetal age, cell passages and time in culture. After 40-60 days it could reach a percentage of 80%. However, after the 15th week of gestation after several passages the percentage of positive cells tended to decrease. These results applied to *in toto* cultures. When the different brain regions were cultured separately, discrepancies in the percentage of positive cells among regions were detected being the frontal cortex always the lowest in Ia-positive cell content. Also the distribution of the antigen varied with time. As shown in Fig. 1, at earlier stages Ia-positive cells were round-shaped, negative for GFA-P and the antigen was detectable on the cell surface. Later, as shown in Fig. 2, the antigen was predominantly located in flat, process-bearing GFA-P+ cells and it was detectable both on the surface (a) and in the cytoplasm (b). However, there were still Ia-positive cells which were negative for GFA-P. On the other hand, not all the GFA-P^+ astrocytes bore Ia antigens. Double staining with neurofilament antibody failed to show the presence of Ia^+ neurons.

DISCUSSION

Our data provide evidence that brain cells of very young fetuses can spontaneously express HLA-DR after a very brief period in culture. Since these HLA-DR^+ cells did not show other specific labeling, such as GFA-P, their origin remained unknown. However, our cultures have been shown to be enriched in neurons, astrocytes and their precursors.[12] Thus, it is likely that they were young astrocytes which did not yet express GFA-P. In fact, our cultures also

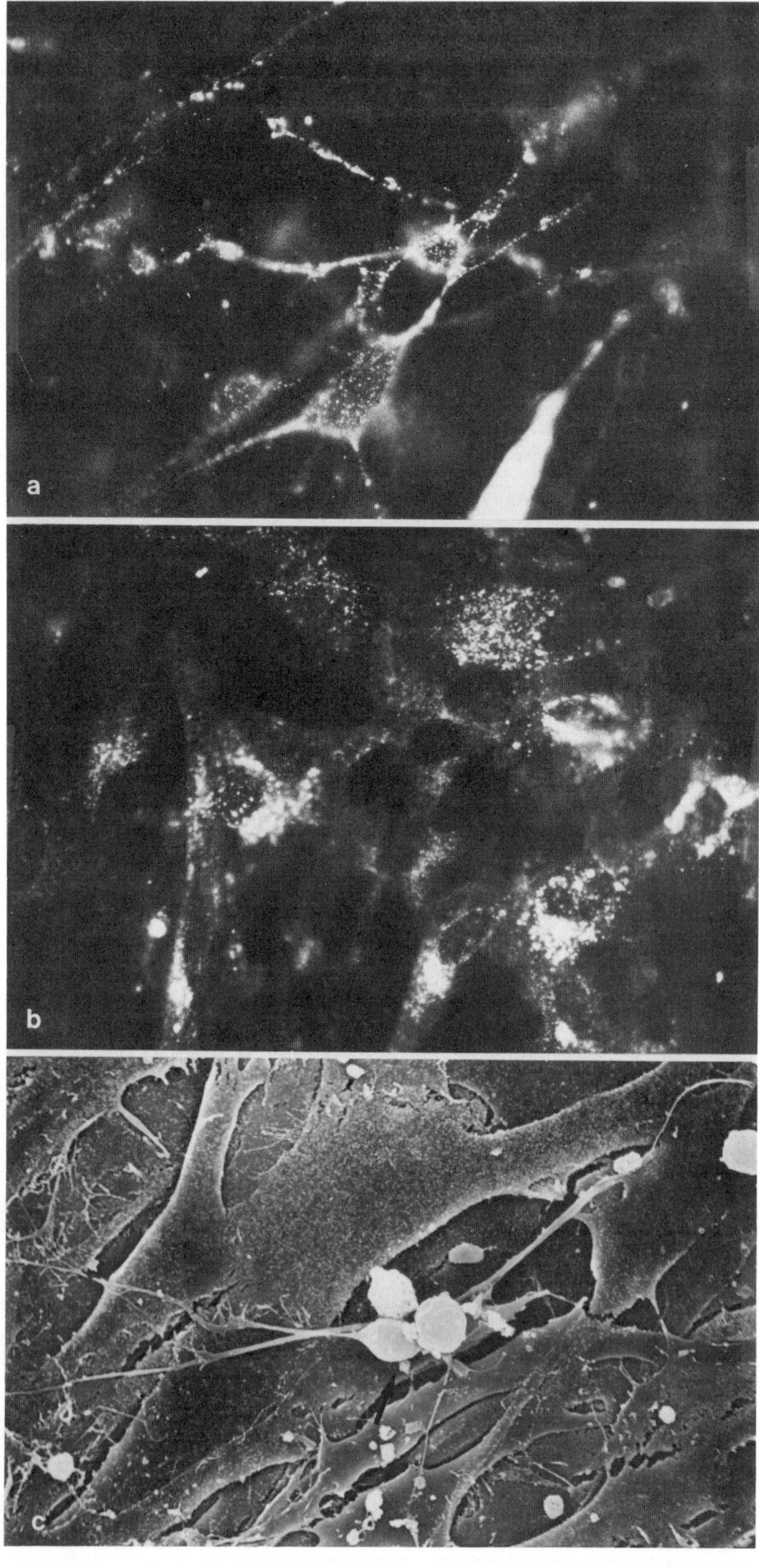
a
b
c

contain A2B5$^+$ cells, ie, the common precursor for oligodendrocytes and type II astrocytes.[12]

Several authors have reported the presence of Ia-positive astrocytes in fetal cultures,[7,8] fetal total brain,[2,13] adult brain[14] and adult brain cultures.[5] However, the percentage of Ia+ cells was extremely variable among authors' reports. In culture, the expression of Ia reached the highest values. Kim et al[5] reported the presence of up to 24% of GFA-P$^+$ astrocytes expressing HLA-DR in human adult brain cultures. On the other hand, Pulver et al[7] reported that in brain cultures from a single 20-week-old fetus there were two cell lines. One of those never expressed HLA-DR, the second one spontaneously expressed the antigen in the proportion of 25%, but lost its capacity with *in vitro* passages. Our earlier cultures showed the opposite phenomenon, since passages increased HLA-DR expression. These observations are also confirmed by Mauerhoff et al[8] who also observed the gradual, spontaneous appearance of Ia positivity in type II astrocytes, which reached the percentage of 50% after 20 days in culture. However, our data add some significant informations to these studies. We were able to show that even at 8th week of gestation there were cells capable to express Ia, even if they did not express GFA-P and were not morphologically differentiated. Moreover, we provide evidence that there are indeed differences in brain regions. Thus, the discrepancies in the findings reported by different authors could simply be due to different sources of brain cells.

This is indeed a very important observation. There is increasing evidence that astrocytes belong to different subtypes.[15,16] Thus, it can be speculated that Ia expression capability is restricted to one or two but not to all astrocyte subtypes, and may correlate with their different functions. It has been reported by several authors that astrocytes can act as macrophages under certain circumstances[17] as well as antigen-presenting cells.[18] Thus, it can be speculated that interferon, instead of just stimulating the expression of Ia antigen, might act as growth factor inducing the proliferation of a specific cell type able to spontaneously express Ia antigen. This possibility seems to us more likely than assuming the expression of class II antigens being constantly suppressed by unidentified humoral or locally produced mediators.

Of course, we cannot exclude that the abundant debris contained in cultures could have triggered the expression of class II, as has been previously suggested.[8] However, since the expression was increased in long term cultures and the expression occurred a few days after the passage, this phenomenon might have an influence at the beginning, but not after a few weeks.

Moreover, Janossy et al[19] described in cultures of human fetuses two macrophage-like accessory cell populations with separate ontogeny, one of which expressing at percentage increasing with time in culture high amounts of MHC-class II and the other not. A similar phenomenon could occur in astrocytes.

Fig. 2. HLA-DR expression in human fetal brain cultures at Day 30 in vitro. The antigen is present in flat, process-bearing cells, which are mostly positive for GFA-P (type II astrocytes). (a) When cells were incubated unfixed, the antigen was clearly distributed on the surface of cell bodies and processes (arrows). (b) When cells were prefixed with methanol and Triton X-100 was added to the buffer, the antigen was clearly detectable also in the cytoplasm (arrows). Magnification = X 500. (c) Immunocytochemical staining at SEM shows the presence of HLA-DR on the surface of some glial cells (white arrows) whereas neurons (black arrow) are negative. Magnification = X 4,710.

ACKNOWLEDGEMENTS

This research was supported by MPI Grant to F.G. and Regione Autonoma Sardegna (Assessorato Igiene e Sanità).

REFERENCES

1. K. A. Williams, D. N. J. Hart, J. W. Fabre, and P. J. Morris, Distribution and quantitation of HLA-ABC and DR (Ia) antigens of human kidney and other tissues, *Transplantation*, 29:274-279 (1980).
2. P. G. Natali, G. De Martino, V. Quaranta, M. R. Nicotra, F. Frezza, A. M. Pellegnino, and S. Ferrone, Expression of Ia-like antigens in normal human non-lymphoid tissues, *Transplantation*, 31:75-78 (1981).
3. M. R. Hirsch, J. Wietzerbin, M. Pierres, and C. Goridis, Expression of Ia antigens by cultured astrocytes treated with gamma-interferon, *Neurosci.Lett.*, 41:199-204 (1983).
4. U. Traugott, L. C. Scheinberg, and C. S. Raine, On the presence of Ia-positive endothelial cells and astrocytes in multiple sclerosis lesions and its relevance to antigen presentation, *J.Neuroimmunol.*, 8:1-14 (1985).
5. S. U. Kim, G. Moretto, and D. H. Shin, Expression of Ia antigens on the surface of human oligodenocytes and astrocytes in culture, *J. Neuroimmunol.*, 10:141-149 (1985).
6. G. H. W Wong, P. F. Bartlett, I. Clark-Lewis, P. Batty, and J. W. Schrader, Inducible expression of H-2 and Ia antigens on brain cells, *Nature*, 310:688-691 (1984).
7. M. Pulver, S. Carrell, J. P. Mach, and De Tribolet, Cultured human fetal astrocytes can be induced by interferon-gamma to express HLA-DR, *J. Neuroimmunol.*, 14:123-133 (1987).
8. T. Mauerhoff, R. Pujol-Borrell, R. Mirakian, and G. F. Bottazzo, Differential expression and regulation of major histocompatibility complex (MHC) products in neural and glial cells of the human fetal brain, *J.Neuroimmunol.*, 18:271-289 (1988).
9. P. F. Bartlett, Pluripotential hemopoietic stem cell in adult mouse brain, *Proc.Nat.Acad.Sci.* USA, 79:2722-2725 (1982).
10. W. R. Walker, R. H. J. Beelen, P. J. Buckley S. L. Melvin, and S. E. Yen, Some fixation reagents reduce or abolish the detectability of Ia antigen and HLA-DR on cells, *J.Immunol.Meth.*, 67:89-99 (1984).
11. B. Pettmann, J. C. Louis, and M. Sensenbrenner, Morphological and biochemical maturation of neurones cultured in the absence of glial cells, Nature, 281:378-380 (1979).
12. M. G. Ennas, S. Torelli, V. Sogos, C. Marcello, A. Riva, and F. Gremo, Immunocompetent-like cells in human fetal brain cultures, in this volume.
13. M. Gerosa, M. Chilosi, A. Ianucci, M. Montagna, G. C. Adrighetto, G. Stevanoni, and G. Tridente, Immunohistochemical characterization of Ia-DR-positive cells in normal human brains and gliomas, *J.Neuro-Oncol.*, 2:272 (1984).
14. S. L. Hauser, A. K. Bhan, F. H. Gilles, C. J. Hoban, E. L. Reinherz, S. F. Schlossman, and H. L. Weiner, Immunohistochemical staining of human brain with monoclonal antibodies that identify lymphocytes, monocytes and Ia antigen, *J.Neuroimmunol.*, 5:197-205 (1983).
15. M. C. Raff, E. R. Abney, J. Cohen, R. Lindsay, and M. Noble, Two types of astrocytes in cultures of developing rat white matter: differences in morphology, surface gangliosides and growth characteristics, *J.Neurosci.*, 3:1289 (1983).
16. J. G. Dickson, T. P. Flanigan, J. T. Kenshead, P. Doherty, and P. S. Walsh, Identification of cell surface antigens present exclusively on a subpopulation of astrocytes in human fetal brain cultures, *J.Neuroimmunol.*, 5:111-123 (1983).

17. H. Kusaka, A. Hirano, M. B. Borstein, G. R. W. Moore, and C. S. Raine, Transformation of cells in organotypic cultures of mouse spinal cord, *J.Neurol.Sci.*, 72:77-89 (1986).
18. W. Fierz, B. Endler, K. Reske, H. Wekerle, and A. Fontana, Astrocytes as antigen-presenting cells. Induction of Ia antigen expression on astrocytes by T cells via immuno-interferon and its effect on antigen presentation, *J.Immunol.*, 134:3785-3793 (1985).
19. G. Janossy, M. Bofil, L. W. Pulter, E. Rawling, G. D. Burford, C. Navarette, A. Ziegler, and E. Kelemen, Separate ontogeny of two macrophage-like accessory cell populations in the human fetus, *J.Immunol.*, 136:4354-4361 (1986).

THE EXPRESSION OF Ia ANTIGEN IN THE COURSE OF ACUTE AND RELAPSING EXPERIMENTAL ALLERGIC ENCEPHALOMYELITIS IN THE LEWIS RAT

Christine D. Dijkstra, C.H. Polman*, A. Kreike, C.J.A. De Groot, J.C. Koetsier* and T. Sminia

Department of Cell Biology and *Neurology
Vrije Universiteit, PO Box 7161
1007 MC Amsterdam, The Netherlands

INTRODUCTION

Acute experimental allergic encephalomyelitis (AEAE) can be induced in Lewis rats by immunization with nervous tissue or myelin basic protein (MBP) in Freud's complete adjuvant.[1] The course of the disease is usually monophasic and animals recover without remnant clinical signs. After treatment with low doses of cyclosporin A in the initial phase of the disease, the course of the disease becomes relapsing-remitting (CREAE).[2]

The number of indications for the fact that the expression of MHC Class II antigens plays an important role in the pathogenesis of experimental allergic encephalomyelitis (EAE) increases. Class II antigens, or Ia antigens, are present on the surface of B cells and antigen presenting dendritic cells, and can be induced on a variety of other cells, both blood borne and non-haematogenic cells.[3] Activated T cells and their products, such as γ-interferon, contribute to this induction of Ia antigen on various cell types.[4]

Under pathological conditions, two major types of cells can express Ia antigen in the central nervous system (CNS), being the infiltrated blood borne cells, such as lymphocytes and macrophages,[5,6] and the supportive tissue of the CNS itself, ie, the vascular endothelium and the neuroglial cells.[7-10] However, there are apparent discrepancies among several studies on role of the expression of Ia antigen in EAE and other demyelinating diseases of the CNS. Some authors claim that the expression of Ia antigen on glial cells is crucial for the induction of the disease, whereas others claim such a role for Ia antigen on endothelial cells.

Whether rat endothelial cells are positive for Ia antigens is a matter of discussion.[7,8,11] Because of the relevance of this phenomenon for the discussion on the pathogenic factors in demyelinating diseases, we studied the expression of Ia antigen on the different cell types in the CNS of Lewis rats in the course of acute and chronic relapsing EAE.

MATERIALS AND METHODS

Animals

Lewis rats (180-200 g) were obtained from the Zentralinstitut Fir Versuchstierzucht (ZFV, Hannover, FRC) and kept under routine laboratory conditions.

Induction of EAE

Acute EAE (AEAE) was induced by a single inoculation of 50 µl guinea pit spinal cord homogenate GPSC), mixed with complete Freunds adjuvant.[5] Chronic relapsing EAE (CREAE) was induced by administration of a low dose of cyclosporin A (Sandoz; 2 mg/kg body weight) every other day from Day O till Day 22 after the inoculation with GPSC.2

CNS tissue was obtained from animals with AEAE at the following stages: Day 8, 10, 11, 12, 14, 15, 24, and 50 after inoculation with GPSC, and from animals with CREAE at Day 10, 11, 12 and 50 after inoculation with GPSC. At least two animals were used for each stage. CNS tissue (medulla oblongata, cerebellum, cerebrum) was frozen in liquid nitrogen. An additional group of animals was used for perfusion fixation on Day 14, 18, 21 and 32 after induction of AEAE, to allow precise judgement of Ia expression of endothelial cells.

Immunohistochemistry on Frozen Tissue

Cryostat sections were fixed in acetone and stained for Ia antigen in a two-step immunoperoxidase method using mouse monoclonal antibody to rat Ia antigen (OX4, Serotex, UK) in the first step, and a peroxidase conjugated rabbit-anti-mouse IgG (RAM/PO, Dakopatta, Denmark) in the second step. After incubation with the first antibody for 60 min, the slides were rinsed thoroughly in PBS and incubated with RAM/PO in PBS/BSA and 1% normal rat serum. Slides were washed again thoroughly in PBS and peroxidase activity was demonstrated with 0.5 mg/ml 3,3'-diaminebenzidine-tetrahydrochloride (DAB, Sigma, St Louis, MO, USA) in 0.05 M Tris-HC1 buffer, pH 7.6 containing 0.02% H_2O_2 for 10 min. Slides were then washed in saline, incubated in saline with 0.5% $CuSo^4$ for 5 min, and washed again in saline. Sections were lightly counterstained with haematoxylin, dehydrated and mounted in Entellan (Merck, FRG).

Immunohistochemistry for Plastic Embedded Tissue

After perfusion fixation[12] with PLP12, the central nervous tissue was dissected and immersed in the same fixative for 4 hours. Slices of approximately 100 m thickness were prepared on a Vibratome. After washing in 0.001 M phosphate buffered saline (PBS, pH 7.4) these slices were subsequently incubated with monoclonal OX4 (mouse anti-rat Ia antigen) overnight, in peroxidase conjugated rabbit-anti-mouse IgG overnight and 3,3'-diaminobenzidine-tetrahydrochloride with 0.02% H_2O_2 for 60 min. After each incubation step, the slices were washed thoroughly with PBS. The slices were postfixed in 1% osmium tetroxide in PBS for 60 min on ice, dehydrated in ethanol and propylenoxide and embedded in araldite. Hardening of the slices in araldite occurred at 60°C between sheets of plastic and two copper bars to keep the slices flat. Under the microscope the slices were judged and areas with infiltrates were selected and trimmed out, embedded in araldite again. Semithin sections of 1 µm thickness were cut with a glass knife of a Reichert ultramicrotome and counterstained with toluidin blue for light microscopy examination.

RESULTS

Clinical Signs

All animals developed clinical signs, except of course those that were sacrificed before the onset of clinical signs. Clinical signs became apparent at Day 11 in most of the animals, always preceded by loss of body weight. Of the animals treated with low dose CsA to induce chronic relapsing EAE and used to study at a late stage (Day 50), five out of eight developed one or more relapses. None of the animals killed at Day 50 were clinically ill at that stage.

Ia Expression in the Course of AEAE and CREAE

On Day 10 after immunization, just before the onset of clinical signs, the first Ia expression in the CNS parenchyma was observed in the medulla oblongata. On Day 11 after immunization, Ia expression starts in the cerebellum and the optical nerve, increasing gradually till reaching the intensity of the medulla oblongata on Day 14. The expression of Ia antigen in the cerebrum reaches substantial levels on Day 15. We did not observe any differences between the CsA treated CREAE animals and the animals with AEAE in these early stages. In general, the expression of Ia antigen is the strongest in the medulla oblongata, where also the number of infiltrates is the highest.

During the clinical phase and the early days after disappearance of the clinical signs (from Day 11 till Day 24) a gradually increasing expression of Ia antigen on different types of cells was observed. Even 14 days after disappearance of the clinical signs, the rate of Ia expression was considerably higher than at Day 10, just before the appearance of clinical signs.

Ia-antigen was expressed on infiltrated cells around blood vessels (Cf[5]). Furthermore glial cells appeared to be positive for Ia antigen, in particular the glial cells that were located near those blood vessels, that were surrounded by infiltrated T lymphocytes and macrophates. Later after disappearance of the clinical signs at Day 50, macrophages and T cells are still present near blood vessels. Furthermore Ia-positive glial cells were still observed dispersed throughout the white matter, but the number, as well as the staining intensity of the Ia positive glial cells, had decreased considerably as compared to Day 24 in animals with AEAE.

In the animals treated with low dose cyclosporin A, the expression of Ia in the white matter was enormous at Day 50 after immunization, in contrast to the situation in acute EAE at that stage. Ia expression was observed on macrophages and T cells in the perivascular infiltrates but also on glial cells.

Ia Expression on Endothelial Cells

On cryostat sections, the accumulation of blood borne cells in and near the blood vessel wall made it difficult to judge whether the endothelium itself was positive for Ia antigen. In heavily infiltrated blood vessels, the endothelial cells lining the lumen often seemed to be positive. In less infiltrated blood vessels, in particular venules, it was possible to observe that elongated, spindle-shaped cells at the parenchymal side of the endothelium (pericytes) incidentally showed Ia positivity.

Even on semithin sections of plastic embedded material, the lower magnifications hardly allowed us to judge whether endothelial cells were positive or not. At higher magnifications it became obvious that not the endothelial cells, but large cells with irregular cell processes in the vessel wall exhibited strong Ia expression. These cells were at the luminal side of the blood vessel always covered by a layer of endothelial cytoplasm that was negative for Ia antigen. The Ia positive cells in the vessel wall were sometimes in contact with cells with similar features in the CNS parenchyma surrounding the blood vessel. At some places and particularly in vessels with infiltrates, the endothelium was higher and the nuclei less condensed than in normal endothelium.

DISCUSSION

The present study shows that the Ia expression in the CNS starts at a relatively late stage in the course of EAE, just before the onset of the clinical signs. In the early stages predominantly blood borne cells, T lymphocytes and macrophages express Ia antigen, indicating that the vast majority of these cells are in a state of activation. Somewhat later, also glial cells in the CNS parenchyma become Ia positive.

We never observed any Ia expression on endothelial cells in the CNS, certainly not prior to the infiltration of lymphocytes and macrophages. The Ia positivity of vessel walls appeared by close examination to be due to the presence of Ia positive pericytes that were always covered by a thin layer of Ia negative endothelium. If endothelial cells of the rat brain can be Ia positive at all, which can not be excluded completely by this study, our results show that this is certainly not an early event in EAE. Therefore a role of endothelial Ia expression in the induction of the disease seems unlikely. How the first T cells adhere to and migrate through the blood vessel wall remains to be established. It can not be excluded that class I molecules are involved rather than class II molecules.[14]

We observed that the endothelial cells of those blood vessels that were infiltrated by lymphocytes and macrophages were less flat and had a bigger, less condensed nucleus that do normal endothelium. These findings suggest a differentiation of endothelial cells in the direction of so-called high endothelial venules (HEV). These HEV normally occur in peripheral lymphoid organs and play an important role in the homing of lymphocytes through more or less specific receptors.[15] Whether the venules in the CNS infiltrates play a similar role remains to be established.

CONCLUSIONS

The late onset of Ia expression and the persistence, even increase, after the disappearance of the clinical signs, do not favor a role for CNS Ia expression in the induction of the disease but rather suggest a role in the regulation of the disease.

We never observed Ia positive endothelial cells; a role for endothelial cells in the induction of EAE therefore seems unlikely.

REFERENCES

1. C. S. Raine, Experimental allergic encephalomyelitis and experimental allergic neuritis, in: 'Demyelinating Diseases,' J.C. Koetsier, ed., 'Handbook of Clinical Neurology,' Vol. 47, (Rev ser 3), P.J. Vinken, G.W. Bruyn, H.L. Klawans, eds., Elsevier, pp. 429-466 (1985).
2. C. H. Polman, I. Matthaei, C.J.A. De Groot, T. Sminia, J.C. Koetsier, C.D. Dijkstra, Low dose cyclosporin A induces relapsing remitting EAE in the Lewis rats, *J.Neuroimmunol.* 17:209-210 (1988).
3. E. R. Unanue, Antigen presenting function of the macrophage, *Ann.Rev.Immunol.* 2:395-428 (1984).
4. J. S. Pober, M.A. Gimbrone, R.S. Cotran, C.S. Reiss, S.J. Burakoff, W. Fierz and K.A. Ault, Ia-expression by vascular endothelium is inducible by activated T cells and by gamma-interferon, *J.Exp.Med.*, 157:1339-1346 (1983).

5. C. H. Polman, C.D. Dijkstra, T. Sminia, J.C. Koetsier, Immunohistological analysis of macrophages in the central nervous system of Lewis rats with AEAE, *J.Neuroimmunol.* 11:215-222 (1986).
6. C. H. Polman, C.D. Dijkstra, C.J.A. De Groot, T. Sminia, J.C. Koetsier, Presence of Ia positive cells in the central nervous system of the rat during various pathological conditions, *Int.Arch.All.Appl.Immunol.* 83:109-111 (1987).
7. J. K. Vass, H. Lassman, H. Wekerle and H.M. Wisniewski, The distribution of Ia antigen in the lesions of rat acute EAE, *Acta Neuropathol,* 70:149-160 (1986).
8. W. F. Hickey, J.A. Cohen, J.B. Burns, A quantitative immunohisto chemical comparison of actively versus adoptively induced experimental allergic encephalomyelitis in the Lewis rat, *Cellul Immunol,* 109:272-281 (1987).
9. U. Traugott, L.C. Scheinberg, C.S. Raine, On the presence of Ia-positive endothelial cells and astrocytes in MS lesions and its relevance to antigen presentation, *J.Neuroimmunol,* 8:1-14 (1985).
10. R. A. Sobel, J.M. Natale, E.E. Schneeberger, The immunopathology of EAE. An ultrastructural immunocytochemical study of class II MHC molecule expression, *J.Neuropathol* and *Exp. Neurol.*, 46:239-249 (1987).
11. Y. Matsumoto, N. Hara, R. Tanaka and M. Fujiwara, Immunohistochemical analysis of the rat CNS during EAE, with special reference to Ia-positive cells with dendritic morphology, *J.Neuroimmunol,* 12:265-277 (1986).
12. A. J. P. Veerman, E.C. M. Hoefsmit, H. Boeré, Perfusion fixation using a cushioning chamber coupled to a peristaltic pump. *Stain Technology* 49:111-114 (1974).
13. I. W. McLean and P.K. Nakane, Period at-lysine-paraformaldehyde fixative *J Histochem Cytochem,* 22:1077-1085 (1974).
14. Y. Matsumoto and M. Fujiwara, In situ detection of class I and II major histocompatibility complex antigens in the rat central nervous system during experimental allergic encephalomyelitis. An immunohistochemical study, *J.Neuroimmunol,* 12:265-277 (1986).
15. G. Kraal, A.M. Duijvestijn and H.H. Hendriks, The endothelium of the high endothelial venule: a specialized endothelium with unique properties, *Expl.Cell Biol.*, 55:1-10 (1987).

Central Nervous System Diseases and the Immune System

THE USE OF THE POLYMERASE CHAIN REACTION IN THE SEARCH FOR A PERSISTENT VIRUS IN MULTIPLE SCLEROSIS: HTLV-1

Peter Schmid, Andrew Conrad, Diethart Schmid and Wallace W. Tourtellotte

Neurology and Research Services
VAMC W. Los Angeles, Wadsworth Division, Los Angeles and
Department of Neurology
University of California at Los Angeles School of Medicine
Los Angeles, CA, USA

ABSTRACT

The polymerase chain reaction (PCR) is a powerful new technique which if employed correctly can detect single copies of a target sequence. This fact makes PCR an invaluable means by which to finally determine the role viruses may play in multiple sclerosis. However, the PCR technique possesses inherent problems which must be carefully controlled or erroneous results may occur. For example, using the correct methodology we were unable to confirm the presence of HTLV-1 sequence from DNA of multiple sclerosis patients blood mononuclear cells by amplification as reported by Reddy et al.[1] Several reasons for the discrepancies are discussed and suggestions as to how to avoid similar complications while using the PCR technique.

INTRODUCTION

The viral etiology of multiple sclerosis (MS) has been proposed repeatedly for decades. A complete summary of the concepts behind these proposals can be found in the review by Johnson[2] which details the fact that some 13 different and diverse viruses have been implicated in the disease. However, recently several papers have focused attention on the putative role of a single virus, Human T-Cell Lymphoma/Leukemia Virus Type 1 (HTLV-1), in the pathogenisis of MS.[1,3] In Koprowski's 1985 article[3] the author reports the presence of antibodies reactive to HTLV-1 in two populations of MS patients. In contrast, it is important to note that subsequently De Rossi et al, Hauser et al, Karpas et al and Rice et al.[4-7] have all reported consistently negative results. The contradiction is at this time unexplained but may be due to the inherent weaknesses of this indirect form of measurement ie, attempting to demonstrate the virus by determining if patients express antibodies to the virus or by culture techniques.

Fortunately, in the past few years a new, highly sensitive method for detecting extremely low copy numbers of geneomic material, known as the polymerase chain reaction (PCR) nucleic acid amplification technique has been introduced.[8] This technique allows for detection of as little as a single copy of template material and is therefore orders of magnitude more sensitive than any other pre-existing method. It is through the use of this technique that the role of viruses in MS may finally be determined. However, because of the extreme sensitivity and the complexity of this procedure it is filled with inherent difficulties which must be very carefully controlled. Means to overcome these problems will be discussed in an effort to alleviate any ambiguities that surface in the future.

As an example we will discuss a series of PCR experiments we performed in our laboratory to evaluate the potential role of HTLV-1 in MS. In 1989 Reddy et al.[1] employed this new technique and were able to detect nucleic acids from two regions of the HTLV-1 genome in six MS patients and in only one out of 20 controls. This work lead our group to try to duplicate this study on a group of 23 MS patients currently being seen at the Wadsworth VA Hospital. The results of this effort, as well as their explanation, will be detailed in this chapter.

METHODS

All 23 patients had clinically definite or laboratory-supported MS in the chronic progressive phase. The ten controls were healthy normal individuals who worked in the laboratory. Blood (5 ml) was drawn from the cubital veins into vacuum tubes containing EDTA, and mononuclear cells were enriched using Sepracyl. Nucleic acid was then extracted according to the procedure recommended in Perkin Elmer Cetus 'Amplification' News Letter (May 1989, Issue 2). After extractions samples were treated with RNAse A for 2 hours, and then they were phenol extracted and ethanol precipitated. This was done in an effort to ensure that the nucleic acids offered as template for the PCR reaction were primarily DNA. Samples of nucleic acids were then quantitated on a UV spectrophotometer, and 760 ng of this material was used for each PCR reaction. In addition, a ten-fold dilution series of linearized cloned HTLV-1 DNA was made where the final amount of HTLV-1 genome was 4.8×10^{-18} g, this serving as a positive control. All samples in this series were protected by EDTA and 2µg of sheared salmon sperm DNA. The primers were identical in sequence to those presented by Reddy et al.[1] Primers were purified by polyacrylamide gel preparation. The PCR reactions were carried out under the conditions recommended by the manufacturer of the PCR kit (Perkin Elmer Cetus). Each sample was submitted to 35 cycles. For detection of amplified material we performed southern blots on an automated vacuum blot apparatus. DNA in agarose gels was depurinated with HCl, denatured in NaOH and then transferred in a neutral buffer to Duralon (Stratagen) membranes. Detection was done using the new Non-Radioactive DNA Labeling Kit (Boehringer Mannheim).

RESULTS

Experiments using the first set of primers from the *gag* region of HTLV-1 showed extremely high background and several different groups of bands on all 23 patients as well as on all ten controls. (see Figure 1a and b). Annealing temperatures were raised from the normal temperature of 42°C to 55°C and finally up to 62°C in an effort to lower background and nonspecific hybridizations. This had little or no effect. In addition there was marked amplification in blanks that contained only calf thymus DNA or salmon sperm DNA. Dilutions of positive control templates were also positive.

The results from the amplifications using the primers from the *env* region also generated erratic and unexpected results. Amplifications on control dilutions yielded high backgrounds and multiple bands. Only samples of high concentrations (500 ng to 1 µg) of template yielded strong results. (Figure 2a) In our hands with identical reagents (only primers and template were different), PCR has been able to detect other plasmid clones down to 5×10^{-19} g, an amount which represents about five copies of the molecule (Figure 2b). The material from the MS patients showed elevated backgrounds but not strongly positive results.

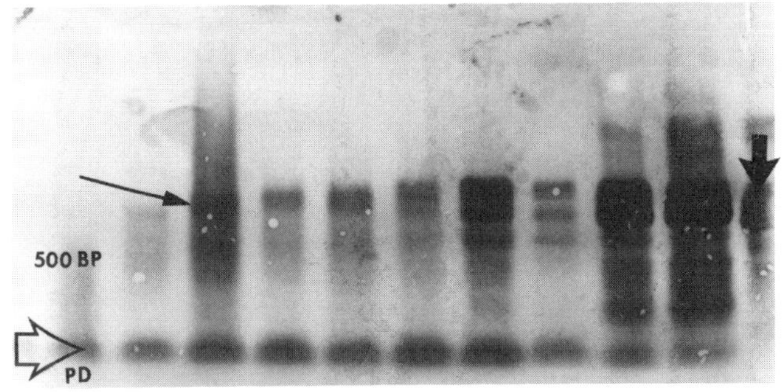

Lane # 1a 2a 3a 4a 5a 6a 7a 8a 9a 10a 11a

Fig. 1(a) Lane 1a. 330 ng of DNA from MS patient #23. Note the position of a 500 base pair band as determined by the control size band in lane 11a. Lane 2a. 660 ng of DNA from MS patient #21. Lane 3a. Blank containing only 2 μg of salmon sperm DNA. Note the nonspecific band slightly larger than 500 base pairs. This band could be misinterpreted for a positive result. Lane 4a. 4.0 x 10^{-15}g of HTLV-1 linearized plasmid in 1 μg of salmon sperm DNA. Lanes 5a-10a are ten-fold increases of HTLV-1 DNA still in 1 μg of salmon sperm DNA. Lane 11a. The 500 base pair marker supplied by Perkin Elmer.
Note: The band indicated by the open arrow marked PD is a band generated from a primer dimer; in other words, from compatible sequences within the two primers annealing and generating this extra band. It is because of nonspecific bands like these that analysis of PCR products should be performed via Southern blotting, and not slot or dot blotting, because Southern blots demonstrate the size of PCR product.

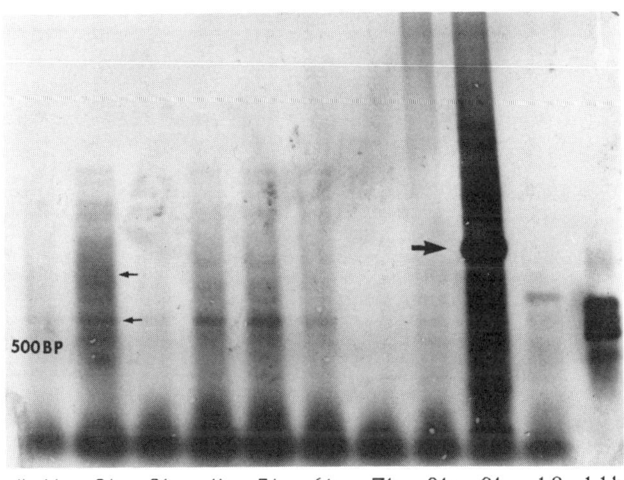

Lane # 1b 2b 3b 4b 5b 6b 7b 8b 9b 10 11b

Fig. 1(b). Lane 1b. 400 ng of DNA from control #3. Lane 2b. 760 ng of DNA from control #2. Note the high background and many bands. Lane 3b. 400 ng from MS patient #19. Lanes 4b-6b. Approximately 700 ng from MS patients #18,17 and 16 respectively. Lanes 7b and 8b. Approximately 400 ng from MS patients 16 and 15. Lane 9b. 2 μg of calf thymus DNA. Note the nonspecific bands and high background. Lane 10b. 4.0 x 10^{-14} g of pure linearized HTLV-1 DNA. Lane 11b. 500 bp control.

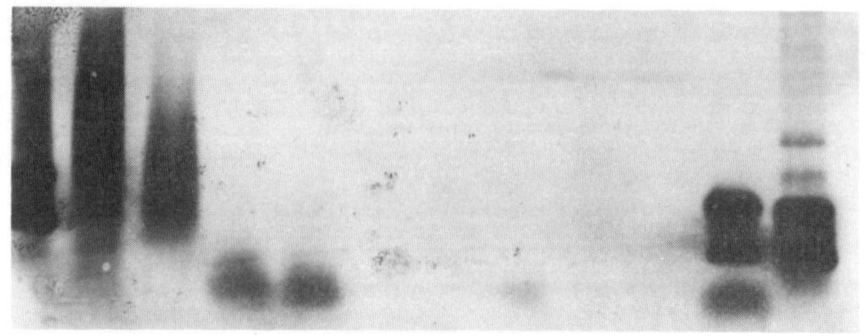

Fig. 2(a). Lane 1a. Pbr322 positive control 350 base pairs. Lane 2a. 0.001 ng of Perkin Elmer control. Lane 3a. 0.00001 ng Perkin Elmer control with 2 μg of salmon sperm DNA. Lane 4a. 4.8×10^{-15} g of linearized HTLV-1 in 300 ng of salmon sperm DNA. Lane 5a. 4.8×10^{-14} g of linearized HTLV-1. Lane 6a. 4.8×10^{-13} g of linearized HTLV-1. Lanes 7a-10a are ten-fold increases in concentration of HTLV-1. Lane 11a. 480 ng of HTLV-1 a 100-fold increase from previous lane. Lane 12a. 1 μg of HTLV-1.

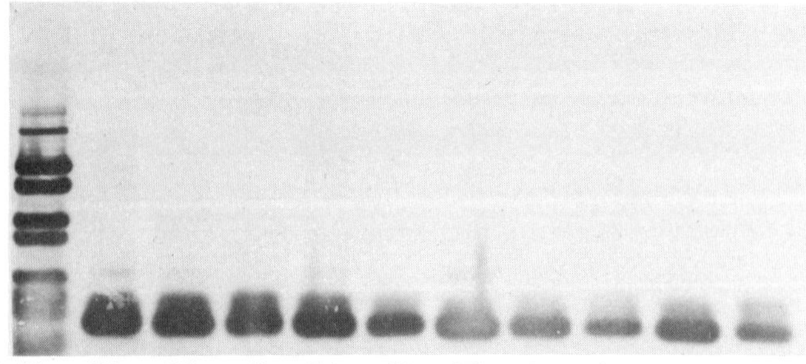

Fig. 2(b). Lane 1b. Boehringer's Markers V which is PBR 322 Hae II digested and used to confirm sizes of PCR products (300 BP). Lane 2b. 50 ng of linearized PBR 322 with 500 ng of calf thymus DNA. Lane 3b. 5 ng PBR 322 in same buffer. Note all samples were diluted in the same Tris buffer which contained 500 ng of calf thymus DNA. Lane 4b. 0.5 ng. Lane 5b. 0.05 ng. Lanes 6b-11b drop by ten-fold increments all the way to 5.0×10^{-18} g.
Note: These primers were selected from the Pbr 322 sequence and are 20 base pairs in length with a 50% G+C content.

DISCUSSION

It is clear that the results we obtained differed dramatically from those obtained by Reddy et al.[1] An explanation of this discrepancy will serve to highlight the fact that if not carefully used, the PCR technique can in fact generate inconsistent results. These inconsistencies can take the form of high backgrounds, nonspecific binding and even false positives.

As demonstrated by Figure 1, use of the gag primers resulted in significant background amplification. The bands demonstrated in this Southern blot were present in material from uninfected cells, calf thymus DNA, as well as in the positive controls and patients. From this information it is reasonable to conclude that there may be homologies with normal endogenous sequences in the genome of higher animals as well as the human genome.

Because of the extremely high G+C content of these primers - 87% for the first primer and 61% for the second primer - they become more likely to generate background. In fact Perkin Elmer Cetus recommends a G+C content of around 50% only. McConlogue et al.[9] details the problem needed to overcome generation of secondary structures and background when using primers with high G+C content. These steps include use of 7-deaza-2'-deoxy GTP mixed with GTP and high annealing temperatures (above 60°C); Reddy and coworkers used the annealing temperature of 55°C and no other special reagents. If possible, when selecting primers it is important to avoid any areas of high G+C content. If the nature of the sequence being investigated leaves no choice then it will be necessary to rigorously control for the possibility of nonspecific binding. The contrast in results may stem from choice of amplification buffers. The buffer they report was at pH 9.3 and contained different salts than did the buffer we used which was suggested by Perkin Elmer Cetus (pH 8.3).

Interestingly, our results are consistent with other published information which suggests that *gag* region of HTLV-1 bears significant homologies (up to 60%) to a human geneomic element which contains provirus-like LTRs and a primer binding site homologous to histidine tRNA.[10] From the sequence of this gene it is possible to locate regions with many seven and eight base pair homologies to the gag primers presented. Of particular interest is the region 2318 and 2458 of the published 5813 base pair sequence. These homologies may be responsible for the high backgrounds we detected. Again, this attests to the importance of careful selection of primers. We suggest that prior to selection of viral primer a detailed investigation into the possibility of homology should be performed.

Further complications existed in the *env* region primers. Upon inspection of published sequences of HTLV-1, we were unable to locate at the position described by Reddy et al any sequence complementary to the env primer sequence they published reportedly to be at base pair 6151. In fact their primer only showed a seven base pair homology with the sequence at this region. The two published sequences of the virus are in agreement at this position.[11,12] The remainder of the primer is unrelated to HTLV-1. This fact greatly reduces the opportunity for this primer to bind adequately under stringent conditions of PCR. To control for errors such as these we suggest examinations of the desired sequence in published references; and if not available to guess at primer sequences is without logic.

The above comments are an example of the problems inherent in the PCR technique and particularly in primer selection we found in attempting to reproduce the results of Reddy et al.[1] The following are some further suggestions which, if employed, will reduce the likelihood of discrepancies arising like the ones described.

1. Select multiple primer pairs or nested primers in the same region and confirm their sequence from multiple sources

2. In order to insure selection of proper target sequences in the viral genome, a careful inspection must be made taking into account the following additional aspects of target sequences: availability of target sequence infor-

mation; avoidance of human homology regions; avoidance of sequence variability in the primer and probe regions; absence of intrastrand complementarity; and presence of proper G+C content.

3. Multiple primer pairs should be used in order to avoid false negatives due to viral mutations as well as confirmational evidence of any positive result.

4. PCR should be done with these primers in control tissues, viral infected cells, uninfected cells, and in cells infected with other viruses. This constitutes an important control sequence for PCR.

5. Additional control experiments for the PCR procedure are especially important for each new set of primers and probes and include the following: serial dilutions of measured quantities of cloned target sequences in carrier DNA, blanks containing high amounts of various carrier DNAs, dilutions of infected cells mixed with uninfected cells and positive control tissues.

Primer selection is just one area from which errors can originate. A second source of problems arises from contamination during the PCR process. Because of the extreme sensitivity of the PCR reaction, great care must be taken to insure that material is not cross contaminated. For example, each experiment needs a positive control in order to rule out the possibility of simple problems like defective reagents. However, this positive control can be the source of a contaminate that if introduced into any sample, even in minute amounts, will generate a false positive result. Some laboratories actually go as far as preparing the positive controls in separate buildings. The following are some steps which have aided us in preventing crosscontamination.

1. Aliquot all reagents into single experiment amounts. In other words, fractionate all buffers, reagents and samples before any positive control material is introduced to the environment. This step will prevent the spread of positive contamination into subsequent experiments.

2. Always discard any aliquot of reagent that has been used, or even opened, during an experiment where positive controls have been amplified. It is important to understand that a post amplified positive control is a extremely rich source of contamination to subsequent experiments and therefore must be kept separate.

3. We suggest that material that has been amplified be further manipulated in a region of the laboratory completely separate from the area used to prepare samples. This means never share tubes, pipet tips, or even water between the two stations.

4. Always scrutinize a positive result by attempting to repeat it on newly acquired independent material.

In conclusion, taking into account the aforementioned errors and the strong tendency of the PCR technique to generate false positives, our observations and precise reading of the Reddy et al.[1] report lead us to the interpretation that their result, ie, HTLV-1 viral nucleic acid sequences were detected in MS blood mononuclear cells and not controls, stemmed from a single source contaminant. Additionally, it is our notion that PCR provides, better than any other method available, a means to determine the presence of viruses in multiple sclerosis brain tissue; but in order to arrive at the correct answer, controls and care must be employed.

ACKNOWLEDGEMENTS

This work was supported in part by the National Multiple Sclerosis Society's Human Neurospecimen Bank (VAMC Wadsworth, Los Angeles, CA, USA) and Merit Review funds from Veterans Administration Central Office.

REFERENCES

1. E.P. Reddy, M. Sandberg-Wollheim, R.V. Mettus, P.E. Ray, E. DeFreitas and H. Koprowski, Amplification and molecular cloning of HTLV-1 sequences from DNA of multiple sclerosis patients, *Science*, 243:529-533 (1989).
2. R.T. Johnson, Viral aspects of multiple sclerosis, in: J.C. Koetsier, Handbook of Clinical Neurology, Elsevier Science Publishers, (1985).
3. H. Koprowski, E.C. DeFreitas, M.E. Harper, M. Sandberg-Wollheim, W.A. Sheremata, M. Robert-Guroff, C.W. Saxinger, M.B. Feinberg, F. Wong-Staal and R.C. Gallo, Multiple sclerosis and human T-cell lymphotropic retroviruses, *Nature*, 318:154-160 (1985).
4. A. De Rossi, P. Gallo, B. Tavolato, L Callegaro and L. Chieco Bianchi, Search for HTLV-1 and LAV/HTLV III antibodies in serum and CSF of multiple sclerosis patients, *Acta Neurol Scand.*, 74:161-164 (1986).
5. S.L. Hauser, C. Aubert, J.S. Burks, C. Keer, O. Lyon-Caen, G. De The & M. Brahic, Analysis of human T lymphotropic virus sequences in multiple sclerosis tissue, *Nature*, 322:176-177 (1986).
6. A. Karpas, U. Kampf, A. Siden & M. Kock, Lack of evidence for involvement of known human retroviruses in MS. *Nature*, 322:177-178 (1986).
7. G. P. A. Rice, H.A. Armstrong, D.E. Bulman, D.W. Paty & G.C. Ebers: Absence of antibody to HTLVI and III in sera of Canadian patients with multiple sclerosis and chronic myelopathy, *Ann.Neurol.* 20:533-534 (1986).
8. R. K. Saiki, D.H. Gelfand, S. Stoffel, S.J. Scharf, R.G. Higuchi, G.T. Horm, K.B. Mullis & H.A. Erlich, Primer-directed enzymatic amplification of DNA with a thermostable DNA polymerase, *Science*, 239:487-491 (1988).
9. L. McConlogue, M.A. D. Brow and M.A. Innis, Structure-independent DNA amplification by PCR using 7-deaza-2'-deoxyguanosine, *Nucleic Acids Research*, 16:9869 (1988).
10. D. L. Mager and J.D. Freeman, Human endogenous retroviruslike genome with Type C *pol* sequences and *gag* sequences related to human T-cell lymphotropic viruses, *J.Virol.* 61/12:4060-4066 (1987).
11. M. Seiki, S. Hattori, Y. Hirayama and M. Yoshida, Human adult T-cell leukemia virus: Complete nucleotide sequence of the provirus genome integrated in leukemia cell DNA. *Proc.Natl.Acad.Sci.*, 80:3618-3622 (1983).
12. K. T. A. Malik, J. Even & A. Karpas, Molecular cloning and complete nucleotide sequence of an adult T cell leukaemia virus/human T cell leukaemia virus type I (ATLV/HTLV-I) isolate of Caribbean Origina: Relationship to other members of the ATLV/HTLV-I subgroup, *J.gen.Virol.*, 69:1695-1710 (1988).

IMMUNOLOGICAL PARAMETERS IN SUBACUTE SCLEROSING PANENCEPHALITIS AND THE EFFECT OF INTRAVENTRICULAR INTERFERON

Carlo Cianchetti, Francesco Muntoni, Annalisa Fratta and Maria Giovanna Marrosu

Istituto di Neuropsichiatria Infantile
Università, via Ospedale 119
I-09124 Cagliari, Italy

Subacute sclerosing panencephalitis (SSPE) is a late, fatal complication of measles infection. From the immunological point of view, it seems to us that two problems are of main interest in SSPE. The first is the individuation of the mechanism leading to the development of SSPE, possibly a defect in the host immune response. The other concerns SSPE therapy: since we have no drug active on RNA viruses, might an enhancement of immune defence improve the course of the disease?

The persistence of measles virus in nervous cells from the time of general infection has been considered related to the early age of measles infection and therefore to a partial ineffectiveness of the immune system.[1] However, the presence of measles-infected cells in peripheral blood (PB) several years after measles infection has been reported also in normal population,[2] demonstrating that virus clearance is not complete in wild measles-infected subjects as well. This datum can support the hypothesis that a small number of measles-infected PB lymphocytes present in normal hosts (considered 'archeology' of a past infection) can escape the immune surveillance system and spread into nervous system just before the clinical onset of SSPE. In this case, a trace of the breakdown of immunological imbalance could be found by studying the SSPE lymphocyte pattern.

STUDY OF LYMPHOCYTE PATTERN

Since 1979 we have been studying cerebrospinal fluid (CSF) and PB lymphocyte subsets using the rosette-forming cell method.[3] Here we report the results of CSF and PB cell study in 20 SSPE patients, using monoclonal antibody (mAb) markers by flow cytometric analysis.

All patients had high antimeasles antibody titer in CSF, with highly increased CSF/serum ratio, and increased IgG index and oligoclonal bands in CSF; clinical and EEG features were at least 'consistent' (according to the terminology of Haddad et al.[4]) with diagnosis of SSPE. Since immunological changes might be different in relation to the phase and rapidity of the evolution, patients were subdivided according to the course: classical (SSPEc) and rapid (SSPEr, when deceased within 3 months after the onset); the four-stage Jabbour's classification[5] was also considered.

Of the 20 patients, 13 were males and seven were females. Mean age at examination was 9 years for SSPEr group (range 4-12), 11 years for SSPEc group (range 3-18) with mean disease duration 3 months (range 15 days-10 months), and 14 years (12-15) for cases in 'vegetative' stage (SSPEv), with mean disease duration of 4 years.

CSF and PB lymphocytes were isolated as previously described.[6] Cells were labelled with T3 (pan-T), T4 (T helper/inducer), T8 (T suppressor/cytotoxic), DR (HLA-DR determinant) and NK (natural-killer) FITC-conjugated mAbs (Ortho Diagnostic System, Raritan, USA) and anti-Tac (T activated cells) FITC-conjugated mAb (Becton-Dickinson, Erembodegen, Belgium). Flow cytometric analysis was performed over at least 100 cells for each determination, using single color fluorescence analysis with a Spectrum III cell sorter (Ortho Diagnostic System, USA). The results are shown in Table 1.

Lymphocyte pattern in SSPE patients showed an increase in the T4/T8 ratio in both CSF and PB, with an increase of DR+ cells in PB in patients with classic course. The most striking alterations occurred in a patient with a very rapid course (decreased 32 days after onset).

P.A., male, born 3.2.1974.
Abrupt onset of SSPE on 8.3.1986 - death on 9.4.1987.

	T3	T4	T8	T4/T8	Antimeasles antibodies
CSF	18	9	10	0.9	1/128
PB	51	24	32	0.8	1/506

The values we found in SSPE patients are similar to those previously reported,[7] although differences from controls are less marked, since in the early report we used controls studied with the indirect immunofluorescence method. Therefore, lymphocyte subset alterations in CSF and PB in SSPE appear to be scanty. However, the immunological role in SSPE could be incident only while the virus is spreading and could escape detection during acclaimed disease status. The shift from low percentages of PB lymphocyte subsets in rapid course patients to normal values observed in vegetative stage subjects may support this hypothesis. The loss of immunological balance could not only be transient, but due more to the activation of the cytokine system than to the increase in CD4/CD8 subset ratio. In our opinion, it is very difficult to believe that the immune system cannot be implicated in the control of virus-infected cells. A common example of this control is furnished by type II HSV infection and, more evidently, by progressive multifocal encephalopathy.

INTRAVENTRICULAR INTERFERON TREATMENT

SSPE treatment has thus far been completely discouraging. The use of isoprenosine prompted several studies; however, no real improvement was found. Recently Panitch et al.[8] reported some improvement with natural alpha interferon (IFN) administered by the intraventricular (iv) route, since IFN hardly crosses the blood-brain barrier. Alpha-IFNs exert their antiviral effect in party by inhibiting the synthesis of viral messenger RNAs and viral specific proteins and in part by enhancing the immune system, especially through natural-killer, lymphocyte killer and macrophage activity. For clinical trials IFNs are available from recombinant DNA technology; in particular, we used alpha-2a IFN (Roferon A, Roche), henceforward referred to simply as IFN.

To date, we have treated four patients with IFN by the iv route. Here we report clinical and immunological changes occurring in two patients during IFN treatment. In the third patient, IV IFN was started when she was in advanced stage 2 after rapid deterioration; no improvement was observed and iv IFN was discontinued after 4 months. A fourth patient has been in therapy only since August 1988, with some improvement being shown.

Table 1. Lymphocyte subsets from SSPE patients and controls

a. Cerebrospinal Fluid

	T3	T4	T8	T4/8	DR	NK
SSPEc	73.6 ± 7.2 (12)	42.5 ± 8.8 (8)	26.8 ± 7.4 (13)	2.0 ± 1.0 (8)	17.0 ± 3.8 (4)	13.0 ± 9.6 (4)
SSPEr	37.3 ± 23.9 (3)	24.6 ± 21.7 (2)	17.0 ± 6.1 (3)	1.5 ± 0.7 (2)		
NID	59.9 ± 23.1 (11)	40.1 ± 15.3 (11)	29.8 ± 12.9 (11)	1.2 ± 0.4 (11)	14.8 ± 13.7 (19)	12.2 ± 20.8 (19)

Significant difference (*t* test): T4/8 SSPEc vs NID $p<.005$

b. Peripheral Blood

	T3	T4	T8	T4/8	DR	NK
SSPEc (13)	61.7 ± 15.7 (13)	44.1 ± 13.2 (13)	21.1 ± 10.0 (13)	2.6 ± 1.7 (10)	21.6 ± 10.3 (6)	19.7 ± 17.3
SSPEv	62.7 ± 7.8 (3)	45.3 ± 15.1 (3)	26.7 ± 6.4 (3)	1.7 ± 0.5 (3)		
SSPEr	44.0 ± 21.5 (4)	33.7 ± 19.4 (3)	25.0 ± 9.6 (3)	1.4 ± 0.6 (3)		
Controls y. (n=20)	64.5 ± 6.5	37.1 ± 5.8	23.8 ± 5.6	1.6 ± 0.5		
Controls ad. (n=350)	66.2 ± 8.1	42.6 ± 7.8	25.6 ± 6.6	1.8 ± 0.7	11.4 ± 3.4	14.3 ± 6.0

Significant differences (*t* test):
T4/8: SSPEc vs controls y. $p<.005$; DR: SSPEc vs controls ad. $p<.001$.

SSPEc: Classic course, stages 1 and 2; SSPEv: Classic course, stage 4 (vegetative); SSPEr: Rapid course, stages 1 and 2; NID: Non-immunological diseases; Controls y. = 4-12 years; controls ad. = 18-50 years.

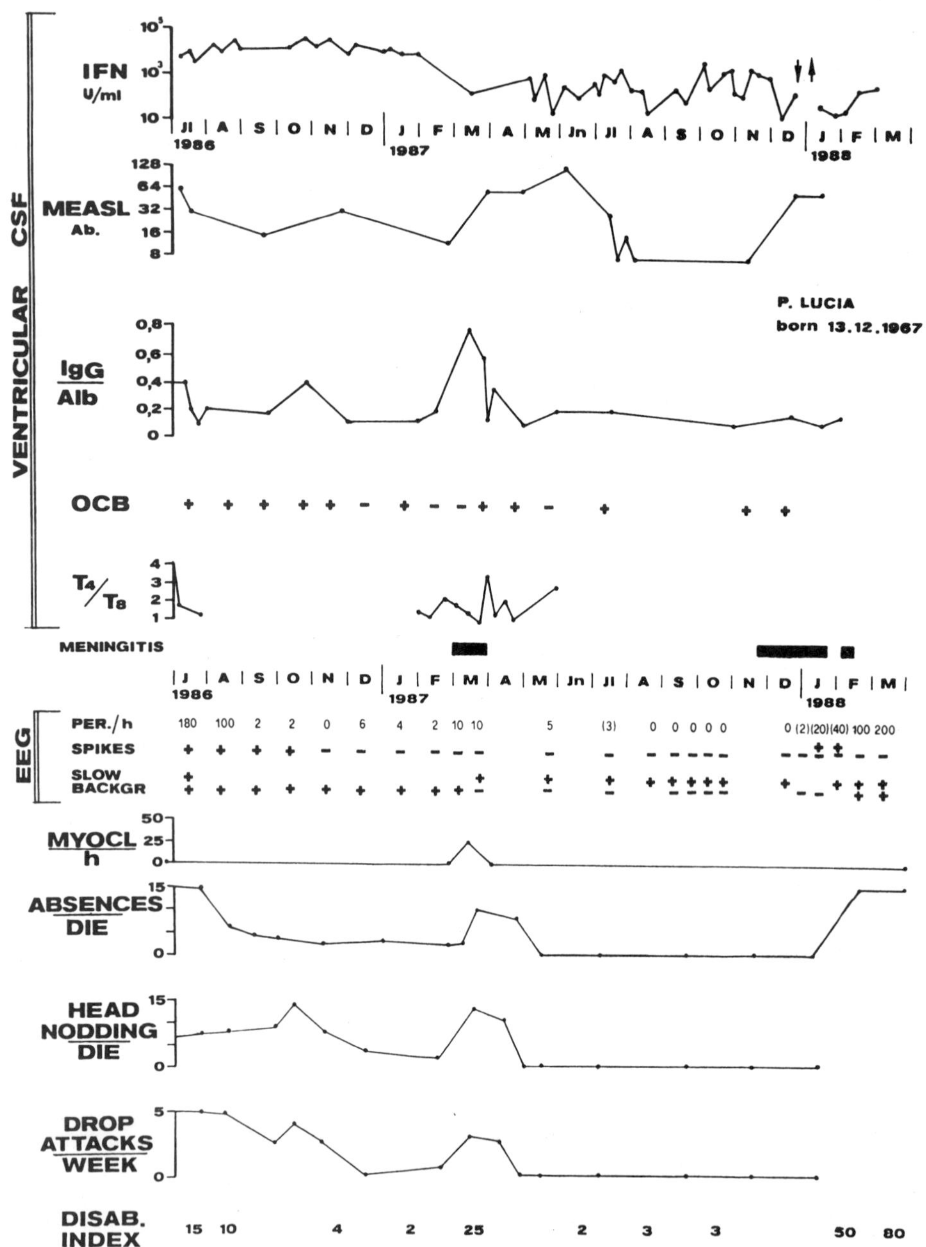

Fig. 1 & 2. Ventricular CSF (upper section) and clinical (lower section) parameters in SSPE patients (No. 1, P. Lucia, female, born 1967; n.2, E. Maddalena, female, born 1971), treated with intraventricular alpha-2A interferon (IFN) (P.L. from July 1986 to March 1988; E.M. from September 1987 to March 1988).

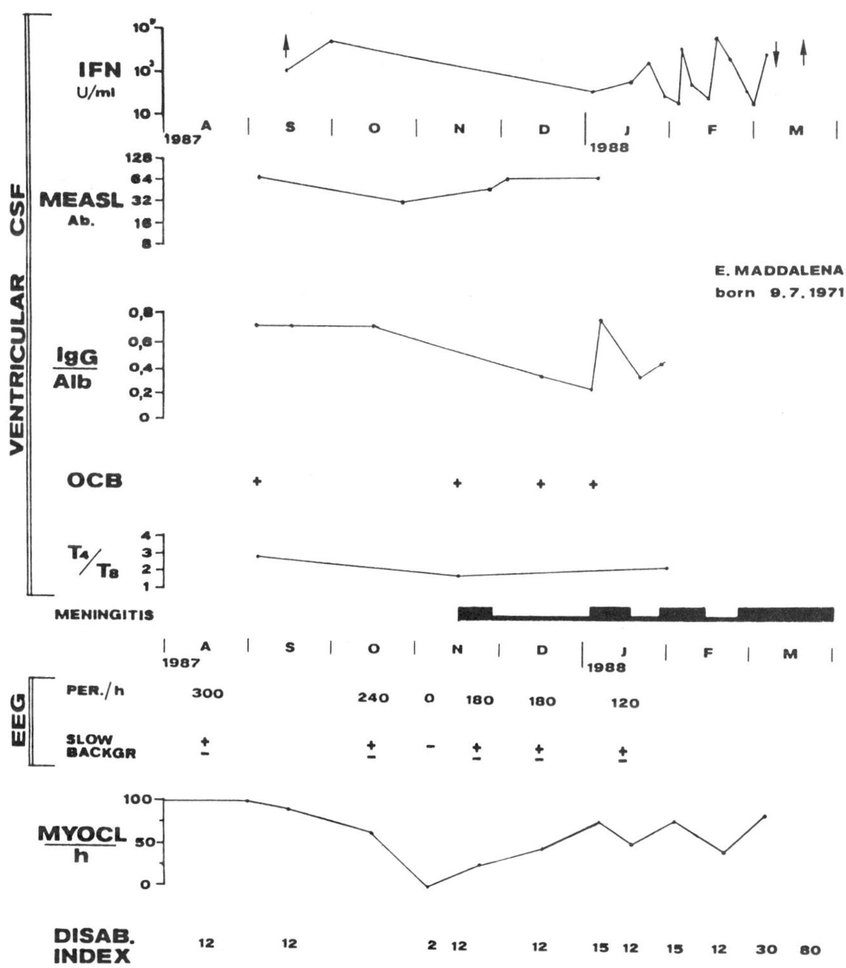

Legend from the top:
IFN U/ml levels dosed (biological assay) before each subsequent IFN administration; arrows indicate stop and restart of drug administration (in this interval IFN levels were not dosed);
measles antibodies titred by immunofluorescent method;
IgG/albumin ratio determined by radial immunodiffusion method;
oligoclonal bands (OCB) detected by polyacrlamide gel isoelectrofocusing;
CD4/CD8 ratio determined by monoclonal antibodies.
Black stripes indicate periods of pyogenic meningitis.
Months indicated by initials.
EEG: Radermecker's periodisms per hour, presence of spikes, presence of slowed background.
Myoclonias per hour; Absences per day; Head noddings per day; Drop attacks per week;
Disability index

In the two patients we describe, IFN was administered iv through Ommaya reservoir at a dose of 1.5 x 10^6 U twice a week; at the same time, 1.5x10^6 U were given subcutaneously (sc), while a further 3x10^6 U sc were given twice a week between the preceding administrations. For a period of about 2 months we tested the effect of an administration of 2.0x10^6 U iv and 1.0x10^6 Usc instead of 1.5 Immunological and clinical data, and their evolution in time, are reported in Figs. 1 and 2.

Clinical parameters (Figs. 1 and 2, lower section) show an improvement in EEG pattern, number of stereotyped attacks (myoclonic jerks, absences, head noddings, drop attacks) and disability index (according to Dyken et al[9]) in both patients. In Case 1 (P. Lucia) in August 1988 (about 13 months after the beginning of IV IFN) bilateral Babinski and EMG signs of 2nd motor neuron involvement (denervation activity, reduced interference, normal nerve conduction) were noted, with slight functional impairment; similar signs in SSPE usually appear only in advanced stages of the disease, after a more diffuse involvement of CNS functions. Therefore we were not able to determine if this was an atypical evolution of the disease or a collateral effect of IV IFN therapy.

Immunological parameters (Figs, 1 and 2, upper section) show an improvement parallel to the clinical improvement. In particular, in ventricular CSF antimeasles antibody titers decreased, IgG/albumin ratio normalized and oligoclonal bands occasionally disappeared. A sudden worsening of all parameters occurred in P. Lucia during an episode of pyogenic meningitis (*Staphylococcus aureus*), with gradual restoration after cure. Due to rebel pyogenic meningitis, in both patients catheter and reservoir were removed, with interruption of iv IFN administration (continued sc at increased doses and frequency); however, within 10-14 days a dramatic worsening occurred; restarting iv IFN after 26 days in P. Lucia and 16 days in E. Maddalena no longer stopped the progressive worsening of the disease and death occurred within a few weeks.

The effect of IFN treatment on the presence of viral RNA in PB lymphocytes was studied in these two patients with a dot-blot hybridization technique, according to Fournier et al.[10] Briefly, PB cells were separated in Ficoll-Hypaque gradient, divided into aliquots containing 1x10^6, 3x10^6, 7x10^6 cells and stored at -80° until required. RNA was isolated using the method described by Cheley and Anderson.[11] As a specific probe for measles virus, an oligonucleotide (nucleotides 1006-1047 of the nucleocapsid protein gene) was synthesized and labelled with ^{32}P. After dot-blot hybridization on nitrocellulose, blots were washed at 58°C and autoradiography was then carried out for 24 hours and 72 hours. Results are shown in Fig. 3.

Positive signals were obtained from a patient who had wild measles infection 10 days before and in two SSPE patients in stage 4 (untreated). In the first SSPE patient treated with IFN (P. Lucia), an increase in signal from stage 1 (during treatment) to stages 2 and 4 (after IFN administration was stopped) is detected. In the second iv IFN treated SSPE patient (E. Maddalena), there is a decreased signal from the beginning of iv IFN (stage 2) to the following two successive evaluations during progressive clinical amelioration (stage 1). Such data therefore show a parallelism between clinical conditions and the presence of viral RNA in lymphocytes, and suggest that the effectiveness of IFN therapy may be monitorized using this technique.

The effects observed in our two patients during iv IFN treatment are as follows: (1) clinical and EEG improvement, until near normalization; (2) manyfold reduction in anti measles antibody titers in CSF; (3) CSF IgG normalization with reduction of OCB; (4) reduction in viral RNA in lymphocytes; and, conversely, (5) rapid deterioration a few days after withdrawal of iv IFN. All these data suggest the effectiveness of iv IFN therapy. It therefore seem that iv IFN can block or slow the virus proliferation and diffusion in CNS, without however eradicating the infection.

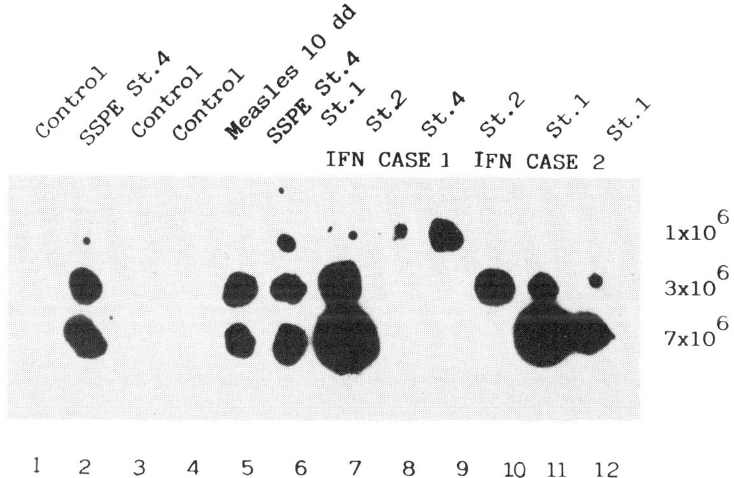

Fig. 3. Dot-blot hybridization of measles virus RNA on PB lymphocytes. On the right side, progressive lymphocyte concentrations blotted on the membrane (0.5×10^6 to 7×10^6) are indicated. Control subject (lane 1) shows negative signals. A case with recent wild measles infection (lane 3) and two untreated cases with SSPE in stage 4 (lanes 2 and 4) show increase of the signal proportional to lymphocyte concentrations. IFN (iv) treated patient n.1 (P.L.) was tested after 2 months of treatment. When she was improved to stage 1 (lane 5), and 1 month (lane 6) and 3 months (lane 7) after iv IFN administration was stopped with subsequent progressive deterioration. At 1×10^6 concentration, a progressive signal increase is detected in lanes 6 and 7 compared to lane 5 (higher concentrations were not serially tested in lanes 6 and 7 due to insufficient lymphocyte availability). The iv IFN treated patient n.2 (E.M.) was tested at the beginning of treatment (lane 8), and 1 (lane 9) and 2 (lane 10) months afterwards, when improvement to stage 1 occurred. At 3×10^6 concentration, a progressive signal decrease is detected in lanes 9 and 10 compared to lane 8 (lower concentrations and higher in lane 8. were not tested due to insufficient lymphocytes availability).

From this experience, it seems to us that iv IFN therapy should be considered in cases with scantly clinical signs (particularly, slight deterioration of higher nervous function) and, possibly, in those not rapidly worsening. It should however be borne in mind that treatment may show collateral effects after a long time, and would probably need be continued for the duration of the patient's lifetime, since interruption of treatment could lead to very rapid and unarrestable progression of the disease.

ACKNOWLEDGMENTS

Dr Antonina Dolei, Professor of Virology, University of Sassari, performed IFN determinations in CSF. Research partly supported by a grant of the Ministry of Public Instruction of Italy.

REFERENCES

1. R. T. Johnson, Viral infections of the nervous system, Raven Press, New York, p. 248 (1982).
2. J. G. Fournier, M. Tardieu, P. Lebon, O. Robain, G. Ponsot, S. Rozenblatt, M. Bouteille, Detection of measles virus RNA in lymphocytes from peripheral blood and brain perivascular infiltrates of patients with subacute sclerosing panecephalitis, *N.Engl.J.Med.*, 5:313-910 (1985).
3. P. E. Manconi, M.G. Marrosu, C. Cianchetti, D. Zaccheo, Surface markers on lymphocytes from human cerebrospinal fluid. II. Altered patterns in subacute sclerosing panecephalitis, *Eur.Neurol.* 6:19-241 (1979).
4. F. S. Haddad, W.S. Risk, J.T. Jabbour, Subacute sclerosing panecephalitis in the Middle East: report of 99 cases, *Ann.Neurol.*, 1:211-217 (1977).
5. J. T. Jabbour, J.H. Garcia, H. Lemmi, J. Ragland, P.A. Duenas, J.L. Sever, Subacute sclerosing panecephalitis: a multidisciplinary study of eight cases, *JAMA*, 207:2248-2254 (1969).
6. M. G. Marrosu, C. Cianchetti, M. Tondi, M.G. Ennas, G. Marrosu, M.R. Murru, P.E. Manconi, Lymphocyte subpopulations in blood and cerebrospinal fluid from patients wtih subacute sclerosing panecephalitis, *Acta Neurol.Scand.*, 67:55-63 (1983).
7. M. G. Marrosu, C. Cianchetti, M.G. Ennas, Lymphocyte subsets at different stages of subacute sclerosing panencephalitis: a study with monoclonal antibodies, *J.Neurol.Neurosurg.Psychiat.*,49:713-715 (1986).
8. H. S. Panitch, J. Gomez-Plascencia, F.H. Norris, K. Cantell, R.A. Smith, Subacute sclerosing panecephalitis: remission after treatment with intraventricular interferon, *Neurology*, 36:562-566 (1986).
9. P. R. Dyken, A. Swift, R.H. Durant, Long-term follow up of patients with subacute sclerosing panencephalitis treated with inosiplex, *Ann.Neurol.*, 11:359-364 (1982).
10. J. G. Fournier, J. Gerfaux, A.M. Joret, P. Lebon, S. Rozenblatt, Subacute sclerosing panecephalitis: detection of measles virus sequences in RNA extracted from circulating lymphocytes, *Br.Med.J.*, 296:684 (1988).
11. S. Cheley, R. Anderson, A reproducible microanalytical method for the detection of specific RNA sequences by dot-blot hybridization, *Analytical Biochemistry*, 137:15-19 (1984).

POSSIBLE IMPLICATIONS OF THE CELLULAR COMPONENT OF THE IMMUNE SYSTEM IN THE PATHOGENESIS OF UNCONVENTIONAL SLOW VIRUS INFECTIONS

Patrizia Casaccia, Anna Ladogana, Carlo Masullo*, Giorgio Macchi* and Maurizio Pocchiari†

Institute of General Pathology and *Institute of Neurology Catholic University, Rome
†Department of Biology, University of Lecce, Lecce, Italy

INTRODUCTION

A group of infectious degenerative disorders of the CNS naturally occurring in animals and man is referred as unconventional slow virus diseases although the etiological agent has yet to be definitively identified. The transmissibility of these disorders, their long latency period, the atypical properties of the infectious agent such as its resistance to nucleases,[101] its inactivation only with high doses of UV[59], or ionizing radiations[2] and its peculiar structure devoid of a detectable nucleic acid, account for the definition given of unconventional slow virus diseases.[48]

Animal diseases include: scrapie, a neurological disease naturally occurring in sheep and goat which was first described in the last century,[105] transmissible mink encephalopathy,[90] chronic wasting disease in deer,[124] and bovine spongiform encephalopathy in cattle.[123]

Related disorders in man are: Creutzfeldt-Jakob disease (CJD), a form of transmissible dementia with its typical and atypical clinical forms,[83] such as Gerstmann-Straussler syndrome;[92] and kuru, a form of endemic cerebellar ataxia of the Fore-speaking population of Papua-New Guinea.[52]

Both kuru[50] and CJD[58] were successfully transmitted to non human primates; CJD was then passaged to cats,[57] to guinea pigs,[84] to hamsters[86] and to mice.[1,85,120] Scrapie was first transmitted from sheep to sheep[30] and from sheep to goats[60] by the inoculation of infected material, and later to small laboratory animals by the injection of suspensions of infected brains from sheep and goats into mice,[22] and then was passaged from mice to rats,[23] and from rats to hamsters.[24]

Despite their infectious nature, those encephalopathies do not show any clinical or pathological sign typical of viral infections such as CSF pleocytosis, or any inflammatory lesion, perivascular cuffing or mononuclear cell infiltration of the cerebral parenchyma.[56]

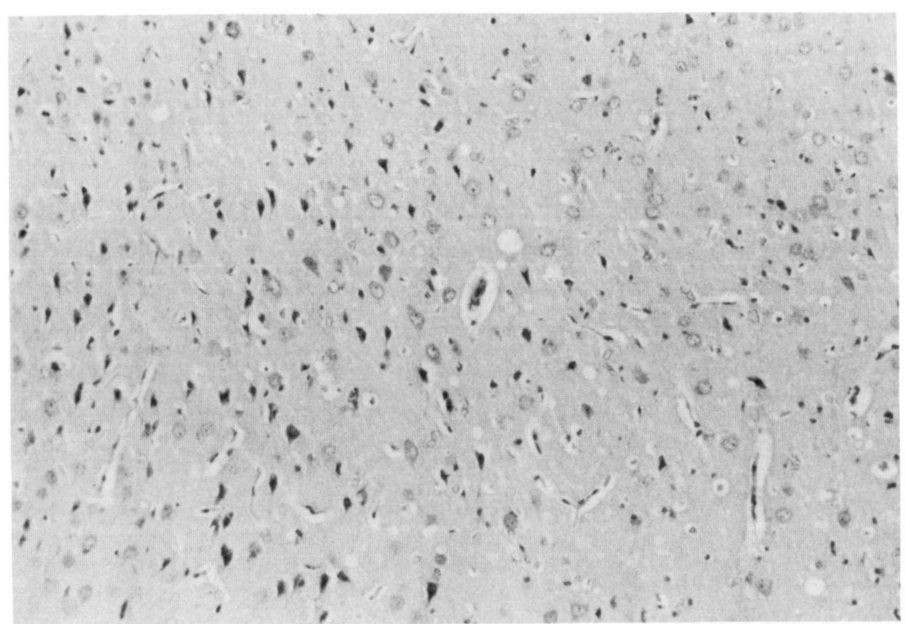

Fig. 1. Spongiosis in cerebral cortex of scrapie-infected hamster. H&E, x 10

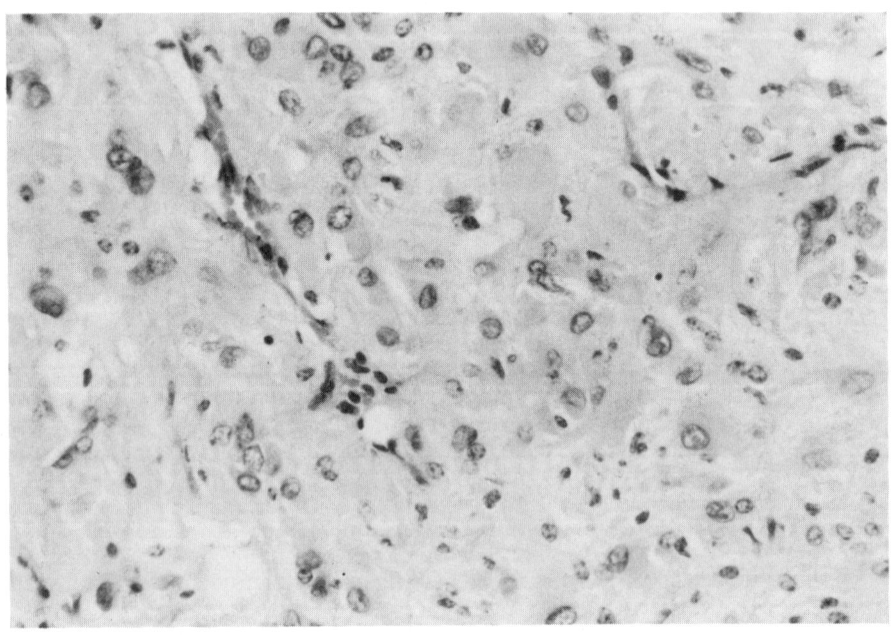

Fig. 2. Astrogliosis in cerebral cortex of scrapie-infected hamster. H&E, x 25

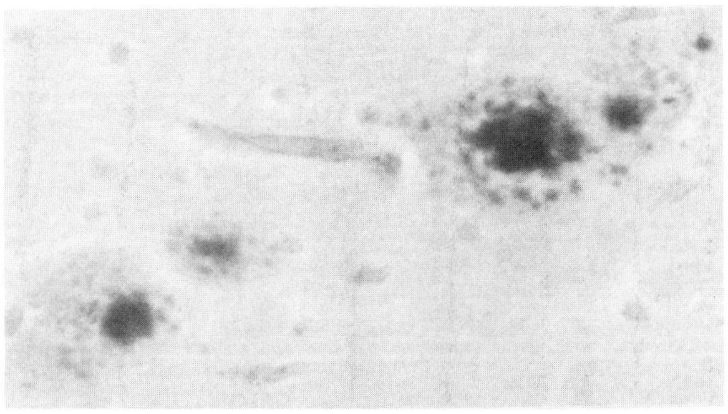

Fig. 3. Amyloid plaques in the cerebellum of a case of CJD.PAS staining, x25

NEUROPATHOLOGY

Neuropathological examinations of brains from affected animals reveal characteristic degenerative changes such as spongiosis (Fig.1), astrogliosis (Fig. 2), amyloidosis (Fig. 3) and a conspicuous although inconstant neuronal loss. Spongiosis is the most typical neuropathological marker of these diseases; in fact it is always present in kuru and CJD patients, except for some cases reported in the literature (for a review see reference 106). Furthermore, the intensity of the vacuolation and its regional distribution defines a different pattern for each virus-mouse strain combination[44] so that any strain of virus can be identified by a typical 'lesion profile'[45] constantly occurring for a particular virus-host combination. Astrogliosis and microgliosis are common findings in experimental scrapie. It has been postulated that these cells may be involved in degradation and processing of amyloidogenetic precursor proteins and play a crucial role in the formation of amyloid plaques.[38,97]

Cerebral amyloidosis has been reported in kuru, in human and experimental CJD, and in natural and in experimental scrapie (for a review see reference 106). Interestingly, the number of amyloid plaques varies with different virus strain-mouse genotype[16] and the incidence of cerebral amyloidosis is higher in animals with a long incubation period.[15] Amyloid in spongiform encephalopathies, however, differs from that of the senile plaques for its biochemical[93] and ultrastructural[99] characteristics.

Negative staining electron microscopy of detergent-treated synaptosomal fractions from scrapie-infected murine brains[99] reveals the presence of infection specific fibrils called SAF (scrapie associated fibrils) that are also found in brain extracts from scrapie infected hamsters, CJD infected mice, guinea pigs and hamsters, and from brain extracts from patients with kuru, CJD and Gerstmann-Straussler syndrome.[98] These structures have a characteristic morphology resembling that of a form of amyloid specific of spongiform encephalopathies: they are formed by two filaments of 4-6 nm in diameter, helically wound around each other with a repeat of 40-90 nm to form rods[98] that stain with Congo Red dye and that show the classical green birefringence with polarized light.[111]

BIOCHEMISTRY

SAF can be so considered as an ultrastructural marker of slow virus infection (Fig. 4), being absent in the brains of patients affected by senile dementia of Alzheimer type and in normal aged controls. Structures with similar morphological and biophysical properties to those of SAF have been termed 'prion rods' by some investigators.[109,111] The major component of SAF is a protein with a

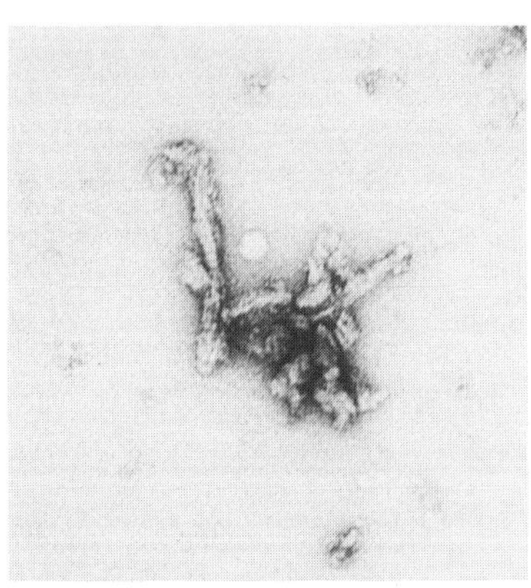

Fig. 4. SAF from scrapie-infected hamster brain. Negative staining, x 60,000

molecular weight of 27-30 kilodaltons (PrP 27-30)[11,39] and with a high tendency to aggregate into filamentous structures.[96] This protein has been purified from infected brains by steps involving sucrose gradient centrifugation, detergent treatment and enzymatic treatments with micrococcal nuclease and proteinase K[109] or by methods of differential centrifugation[40]. Antibodies against PrP 27-30, purified from scrapie-infected animals,[7,41] stain amyloid plaques[5,33], and react with SAF from kuru,[14] scrapie,[7,10] and CJD[8,10,14,88] infected brains.

Much has been so far speculated about the significance of this protein (for review see reference 17). Some authors believe that the protein itself is the infectious agent providing that PrP 27-30 is proportional to the infectivity titre,[95] while others support the theory of an accidental copurification of the atypical virus with the PrP 27-30 with the demonstration of a different kinetics of infectivity and of PrP 27-30 formation[31,32] and with convincing evidence on the separation of infectivity and PrP 27-30 after enzymatic treatment.[87]

The N-terminal sequencing of the PrP 27-30,[110] and the following synthesis of an oligonucleotide probe[104] has made possible the screening of a cDNA library from a scrapie-infected hamster brain and the consequent identification of a clone specific for PrP. A similar cDNA has been also found in mouse infected brain.[25] Further studies have reported the complete sequencing of the PrP gene and the selection of a related cDNA from normal hamster[6,113] and mouse[82] brain. The human PrP gene has been localized on chromosome 20 in man[75,79,112] and its murine homologous on chromosome 2.[117]

The product of this gene is a protein with a low molecular weight of 28 Kda that reaches 33-35 kilodaltons when glycosylated into the cell[12,88,103]; antibodies against PrP 27-30 react either with the pathological protein (PrPsc) or with its normal (PrPc) homologue.[63,100,114] PrPsc differs from PrPc for the sensitivity to protease and detergent treatment. If purified fractions from normal and infected brains undergo enzymatic treatment with proteinase K, PrPc from normal cells is completely digested while PrPsc is cleaved into PrP 27-30 (Fig. 5); furthermore, detergent treatment of scrapie-infected membranes solubilizes PrPc while PrPsc aggregates into rods. Interestingly, scrapie-infected and normal brains contain the same level of PrPc[100] and the levels of mRNA do not change during scrapie infection;[25,104] since PrPc and PrPsc share the same primary structure,[63] the formation of PrPsc must involve some post translational changes, probably a glycosylation or a proteolitic cleavage[64] of the precursor which may yield a conformational change that could account for their different biochemical properties.

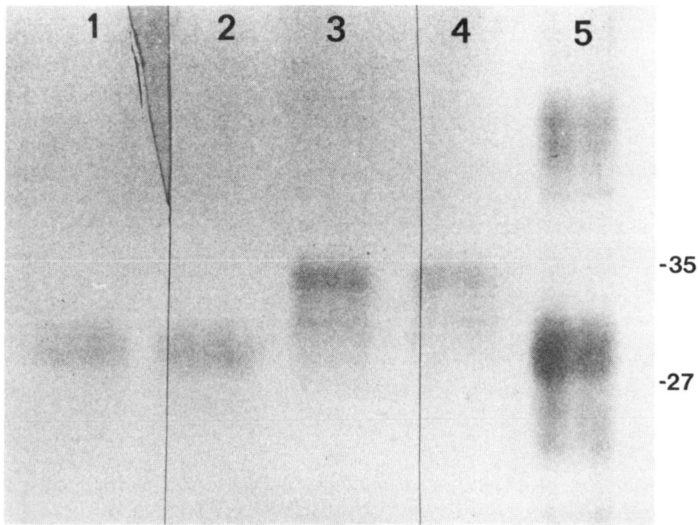

Fig. 5. Western blot analysis of PrP 27-30 protein (purified according to reference 40, lane 5) and of 10% scrapie-infected hamster brain homogenate with (lane 1 and 2) or without (lane 3 and 4) proteinase K treatment (50 μg/ml x 30 min at 37°C). After electrophoresis into a 15% poly acrylamide gel, the proteins have been transferred to nitrocellulose sheets and immunoblots developed using an anti-PrP 27-30 rabbit serum prepared in our laboratory.

IMMUNOLOGY

The expression of the same gene both in normal and in infected cells and the similarities between the two isoforms of PrP leads to speculation about the role of immunological tolerance as a possible cause of the lack of any humoral or cellular response.

In fact early attempts to demonstrate the presence of circulating antibodies in the sera of CJD or kuru patients[51] have failed and the following employment of several immunological techniques on sera from different animal species using different sources of scrapie antigen have not succeeded (for a comprehensive review see reference 67).

The investigation on the cellular response have yielded the same negative results. There is no description of consistent sign of pleocytosis[56] and, apart from a small decrease in the percentage of polymorphonuclear cells reported by Licursi et al[80] and by Dickinson et al,[37] there has been no further evidence of any quantitative change in white blood cells. The lack of infectivity of circulating peripheral lymphocytes[91], the inefficacy of the treatment with antilymphocyte serum[62], and the demonstration of the same clinical course in CBA/N (ie, immunodeficient in the maturation of B lymphocytes),[68] in nude (ie, genetically athymic[102]), in thymectomized (ie, immunodeficient in T lymphocytes[47,94]) in Lasat (ie, genetically athymic and asplenic[102]) or in lethally irradiated mice[94] suggest that mature lymphocytes are not required for scrapie infection. This is further supported by the observation that treatment with immunosuppressive agents like cyclofosfamide[125] or ACTH (Ladogana, Casaccia, Pocchiari, unpublished observation), or with immunomodulators like methisoprinol[108] does not alter the incubation period of scrapie-infected animals.

Table 1. Lymphoid Response After B or T Cell Stimulation in Infected Animals

Mitogen/ Antigen	Cell Stimulated	Lymphoid Response	Reference
LPS	B cell	0 / -	118, 74, 68, 76
PHA	T cell	0 / -	118, 74, 68, 43, 72
ConA	T cell	0	118, 76
Pokeweed	B/T cell	0	118
Sheep red blood cell	B cell	0	26

LPS, Lipopolysaccharide; PHA, phytohemagglutinin; ConA, concanavalin A; 0, normal or -, depressed response.

One possible explanation of the absence of any humoral or cellular response is the impairment of the host immune function caused by the scrapie infection but this theory has not received experimental confirmation, since the agent neither suppresses the antibody production[26,53], nor influences the response of T and B cells to mitogen stimulation[54,55,74,76] even if some authors[118] have reported an inconstant depression of the lymphocytic response to mitogenic stimulation (Table 1). Furthermore, investigation of immunoglobulin content in sera of infected animals have yielded controversial results: while some authors have found an aspecific rise in the IgG content in the serum of sheep with natural[29] and experimental scrapie[28], this rise has not been reported by other workers[119].

Some authors have described the presence of autoantibodies against axonal neurofilaments (Fig.6) in the sera of patients with kuru or with CJD[115] or in that of infected animals[3]. Neurofilaments belong to the class of intermediate filaments and they are composed of a triplet of proteins with molecular weights of about 70, 150, and 200 kDa. The sera from human patients[4,121] and that from infected chimpanzees[122] react mainly with the 150 and 200 kDa components. According to Bahmanyar et al.[4] the infection of splenic cell populations by unconventional slow viruses may account for the production of heterogeneous antibodies showing cross reactivity with neurofilaments; moreover Gajdusek[49] hypothesizes an activation of B-cell clones mediated by the neurofilament proteins released by neurons after a block in the axonal transport. However autoantibodies against neurofilaments can be found also in 11-33% of human subjects affected by other neurological (Parkinson's disease with dementia, Parkinson-dementia complex of Guam, Pick's disease, Alzheimer's dementia) and not neurological diseases[66] and in 10% of normal controls.[4,66,115,121]

If the scrapie agent does not alter the immunological competence of the host then there must be an alternative explanation of the lack of any specific reaction: possibly the scrapie agent is not immunogenic because of its hydrophobicity and membrane binding that may protect it from the exposure of antigenic sites; otherwise it may interact with a cellular component of the host and so escape the host surveillance by inducing a mechanism of immunological tolerance.

GENETIC

There are several experimental data supporting a functional specific interaction between the agent and a host component. The influence of the genetic background on the pathogenesis of scrapie has been studied in mice with different genotypes and inoculated with different strains of virus.[35,36] It has been postulated that a gene called *sinc* (from Scrapie incubation period) controls the length of the disease since s7s7 homozygous mice show a mean incubation

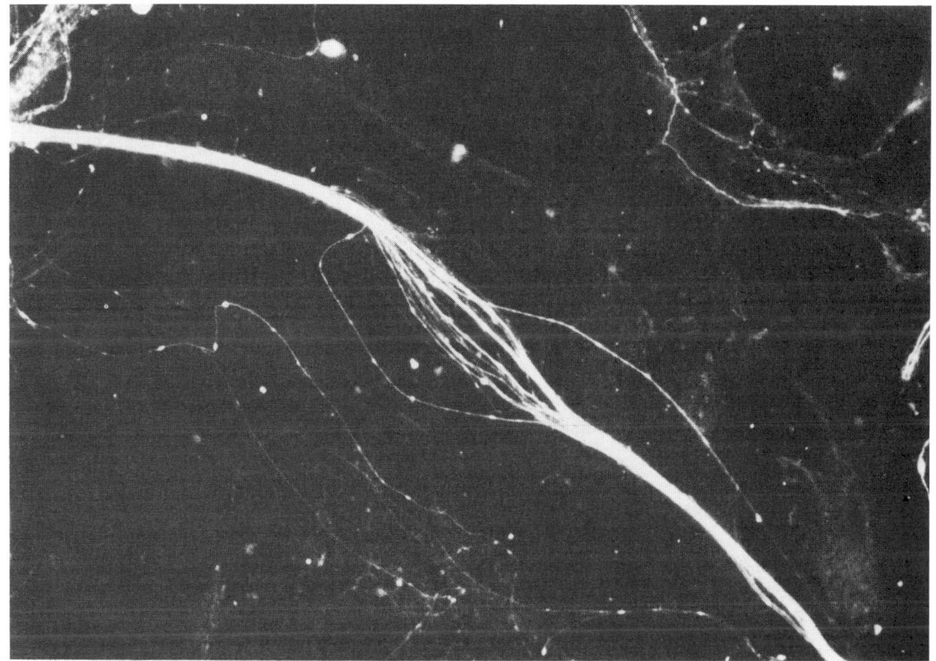

Fig. 6. Mouse central neurons *in vitro* (prepared according to reference 116), immunoreact with serum (921-T, kindly provided by Dr C.J. Gibbs, Jr, National Institutes of Health, Bethesda, USA) from an experimentally CJD-infected African green monkey diluted 1:16 and stain with FITC-conjugated rabbit anti-monkey IgG. This serum contains antibodies against neurofilament[3].

period differing by hundreds of days from that of homozygous p7p7. Such a difference is dependent on the particular strain of virus the mice are injected with, since s7s7 gives shorter values than p7p7 with ME7, while the opposite situation occurs with the 22A. The product of *sinc* is still unknown, however this gene has been localized on the same chromosome as that of PrP suggesting a possible relationship between the products of these two loci.[18,65] Recently the possible involvement of the locus of the major histocompatibility complex in CJD[73] and in scrapie[21] pathogenesis has been postulated. In fact CJD injected mice, carrying the 9 allele of the H-2D subregion of the major histocompatibility complex, show a shorter incubation period than those carrying the d allele. Furthermore, scrapie-infected mice sharing the same genotype (ie, s7s7) but with different alleles at the H-2D locus show interesting differences depending on the inoculation route. SJL (allele s) and NZW (allele z) mice, intracerebrally infected with the ME7 scrapie strain, have shorter incubation period than the C57BL (allele b). SJL mice show the same short incubation period after intraperitoneal injection, while NZW have a great delay of the onset of the disease. The same differences are found also for the infectivity titre since it is lower for NZW ip injected with ME7 (3.7 log) than for SJL (7.1 log) injected with the same agent by the same route, suggesting the possibility that the H-2D locus may act in peripheral infection by different mechanisms involving different alleles.

PATHOGENESIS

Further investigation of scrapie pathogenesis after extraneural inoculation suggests the possibility that the reticulo endothelial system (RES) may play an active role in the infection. Several authors[27,46] have reported an increase in the incubation period of animals splenectomized at different times before or soon after the inoculation by peripheral route, while no difference has been found compared to the sham-operated controls. A similar effect in prolonging the incubation period has been also observed in genetically asplenic Dh mice injected by the intraperitoneal route.[34]

Other lines of evidence that spleen is involved in the extraneural replication of the infectious agent are those reporting the growth of the infectivity titre in spleen since the early phases post inoculation until the appearance of clinical signs. The detection of infectivity in spleen followed by that in the spinal cord and then in the brain have been interpreted as suggestions for a possible neural spread of the agent from the spleen through the splenic nerves to the CNS[70]. Furthermore, some investigators[76,78] reported infectivity specifically associated with the low density fractions of splenic cells, containing lymphoblasts, myeloblasts and macrophages.

The stimulation of macrophage activity in scrapie-infected mice by the injection of vaccinia virus[89] or of a methanol extracted residue of BCG[69] have been resulted in a facilitation of the infection. Both treatments are particularly efficient in shortening the incubation period when they are administered either two hours before or two hours after the inoculation, suggesting a possible early action of macrophages on the initial inoculum. The interaction of the infectious agent with peritoneal macrophages has been further investigated[19] by incubating at different temperatures a 1% suspension of infected brain with these cells or with a tissue culture of kidney cells used as controls. The resulting infectivity is specifically associated with macrophages and it is temperature dependent. The greater amount of infectivity at 37°C rather than at 4°C suggests that the phagocytic activity of mononuclear cells may be involved in their early action on scrapie infection. Since infectivity decreases after prolonged incubation *in vitro*, macrophages do not seem to be a possible site of replication.[20]. The most likely role played by these cells in scrapie pathogenesis, may be that of carriers: they probably remove the agent from the site of inoculation and mobilize it to the first site of replication.

TREATMENT

If this is true then treatment with drugs affecting the cells of the RES will result in a prolongation of the incubation period. It has been reported that polyanions are a class of RES-blockade agents inhibiting the phagolysosome formation either *in vitro*[61] or *in vivo*.[9] Treatment with polyanions such as dextran sulphate 500 (DS-500) has been found to be effective in STU mice[42] or in Compton mice[72] inoculated with scrapie 139A, in C3H mice[43] inoculated with ME7, and in golden Syzian hamsters[77] infected with 263K. DS-500 increases the mean incubation period of scrapie-infected hamsters by 23 days compared to control animals regardless of the dose administered (from 40 to 100 mg/Kg of body weight). Studies with other polyanions (HPA-23) have given the same results.[71,72] We have also demonstrated that another sulphated polyanion, suramin, prolongs the incubation period of scrapie-infected hamsters.[77] Interestingly, treatment with other RES-blockade agents such as silica or trypan blue has no effect. One possible explanation is the shorter half-life of these agents compared to DS-500, which can be detected in mononuclear cells for a period of up to seven months.[42] It is worthy of note the fact that polyanions are effective only in animals inoculated by peripheral routes.

Another drug able to delay the clinical onset of scrapie disease is the polyene antibiotic amphotericin B (AmB). Besides polyanions, AmB is effective both in ip and in ic scrapie-inoculated hamsters.[108] A possible mechanism of action is the interaction of AmB with the scrapie agent on the plasma membrane of the host cells[13] inhibiting its entry into the CNS target cells.[107,108] In ip scrapie-inoculated animals, a further mode of action of AmB may be its effect on mononuclear phagocytes[81] interfering with the mobilization of the infectious agent from the site of injection to the first replication organ(s) (spleen, lymph nodes).

REFERENCES

1. A. L. Abbamondi, G. Di Trapani, M. Pocchiari, A. Sbriccoli, G. Macchi, Problemes de pathologie experimentale dans la maladie de Creutzfeldt-Jakob, *in*: 'Virus non Conventionnels et Affections du Systeme Nerveux Central', L.A. Court, ed., Masson, Paris, pp.309-316 (1983).
2. T. Alper, D.A. Haig, M.C. Clarke, The exceptionally small size of the scrapie agent, *Bioch.Biophys.Res. Commun.*, 22:278-284 (1966).
3. T. Aoki, C.J. Gibbs, Jr., J.Sotelo, D.C. Gajdusek, Heterogeneic autoantibody against neurofilament protein in the sera of animals with experimental kuru and Creutzfeldt-Jakob disease and natural scrapie infection, *Infect.Immun.*, 38:316-324 (1982).
4. S. Bahmanyar, M.C. Moreau-Dubois, P. Brown, F. Cathala, D.C. Gajdusek, Serum antibodies to neurofilament antigens in patients with neurological and other diseases and in healthy controls, *J.Neuroimmunol.*, 5:191-196 (1983).
5. H. Baron, A. Baron-Van Evercooren, J.M. Brucher, Anti-serum to scrapie-associated fibril protein reacts with amyloid plaques in familial transmissible dementia, *J.Neuropathol.Exp.Neurol.*, 47:158-165 (1988).
6. K. Basler, B.Oesch, M. Scott, D. Westaway, M. Walchli, D.F. Groth, M.P. McKinley, S. B. Prusiner, C. Weissmann, Scrapie and cellular Prp isoforms are encoded by the same chromosomal gene, *Cell*, 46:417-428 (1986).
7. P. E. Bendheim, R.A. Barry, S.J. DeArmond, D.P. Stites, S.B. Prusiner, Antibodies to a scrapie prion protein, *Nature*, 310:418-421 (1984).
8. P. E. Bendheim, J.M. Bockman, M.P. McKinley, D.T. Kingsbury, S. B. Prusiner, Scrapie and Creutzfeldt-Jakob disease prion proteins share physical properties and antigenic determinants, *Proc.Natl.Acad.Sci.*USA, 82:997-1001 (1985).
9. N. Bloksma, M.J. de Reuver, J.M.N. Willers, Influence on macrophage functions as a possible basis of immuno-modification by polyanions, *Ann. Immunol.* (Inst.Pasteur), 131 D: 255-265 (1980)
10. L. Bode, M. Pocchiari, H. Gelderblom, H. Diringer, Characterization of antisera against scrapie-associated fibrils (SAF) from affected hamster and cross-reactivity with SAF from scrapie-affected mice and from patients with Creutzfeldt-Jakob disease, *J.Gen.Virol.*, 66:2471-2478 (1985).
11. D. C. Bolton, M.P. McKinley, S.B. Prusiner, Identification of a protein that purifies with the scrapie prion, *Science*, 218:1309-1311 (1982).
12. D. C. Bolton, R.K. Meyer, S.B. Prusiner, Scrapie PrP27-30 is a sialoglycoprotein, *J.Virol.*, 53:596-606 (1985).
13. P. Brown, Biological and chemotherapeutic forays into the field of unconventional viruses, *in*: Targets for the design of antiviral agents, E.De Clerq, R.T. Walker, eds., Plenum Press, New York, pp. 131-137 (1984).
14. P. Brown, M. Coker-Vann, K. Pomeroy, M. Franko, D.M. Asher, C.J. Gibbs, Jr., D.C. Gajdusek, Diagnosis of Creutzfeldt-Jakob disease by Western blot identification of marker protein in human brain tissue, *N.Engl.J.Med.*, 314:547-551 (1986).
15. M. E. Bruce, A.G. Dickinson, Genetic control of amyloid plaque production and incubation period in scrapie-infected mice, *J.Neuropathol. Exp.Neurol.*, 44:285-294 (1985).
16. M. E. Bruce, A.G. Dickinson, H.Fraser, Cerebral amyloidosis in scrapie in the mouse, effect of agent strain and mouse genotype, *Neuropathol. Appl. Neurobiol.*, 2:471-478 (1976).

17. M. Brunori, M.C. Silvestrini, M. Pocchiari, The scrapie agent and the prion hypothesis, *Trends Biochem.Sci.*, 13:309-313 (1988).
18. G. A. Carlson, D.T. Kingsbury, P. Goodman, S. Coleman, S.T. Marshall, S.J. DeArmond, D. Westway, S.B. Prusiner, Prion protein and scrapie incubation time genes are linked, *Cell*, 46:503-511 (1986).
19. R. I. Carp, S.M. Callahan, *In vitro* interaction of scrapie agent and mouse peritoneal macrophages, *Intervirology*, 16:8-13 (1981).
20. R. I. Carp, S.M. Callahan, Effect of mouse peritoneal macrophages on scrapie infectivity during extended *in vitro* incubation, *Intervirology*, 17:201-207 (1982).
21. R. I. Carp, S.M. Callahan, Scrapie incubation periods and end-point titers in mouse strains differing at the H-2D locus, *Intervirology*, 26:85-92 (1986).
22. R. L. Chandler, Encephalopathy in mice produced by inoculation with scrapie brain material, *Lancet*, i:1378-1379 (1961).
23. R. L. Chandler, J.Fisher, Experimental transmission of scrapie to rats, *Lancet*, ii:1165 (1963).
24. R. L. Chandler, B.A. Turfrey, Inoculation of voles, chinese hamsters, gerbils, and guinea pigs with scrapie brain material, *Res.Vet.Sci.*, 13:219-224 (1972).
25. B. Chesebro, R. Race, K. Wehrly, J. Nishio, M. Bloom, D. Lechner, S. Bergstrom, K. Robbins, L. Mayer, J.M. Keith, C. Garon, A. Haase, Identification of scrapie prion protein-specific mRNA in scrapie-infected and uninfected brain, *Nature*, 315:331-333 (1985).
26. M. C. Clarke, The antibody response of scrapie-affected mice to immunisation with sheep red blood cells, *Res.Vet.Sci.*, 9:595-597 (1968).
27. M. C. Clarke, D.A. Haig, Multiplication of scrapie agent in mouse spleen, *Res.Vet.Sci.*, 12:195-197 (1971).
28. S. C. Collis, R.H. Kimberlin, Further studies on changes in immunoglobulin G in the sera and CSF of Herdwick sheep with natural and experimental scrapie, *J.Comp.Path.*, 93:331-338 (1983).
29. S. C. Collis, R.H. Kimberlin, G.C. Millson, Immunoglobulin G concentrations in the sera of Herdwick sheep with natural scrapie, *J.Comp.Path.*, 89:389-396 (1979).
30. J. Cuille, P.L. Chelle, Pathologie animale, la maladie dite tremblant du mouton est-elle inoculable? *C.R.Acad.Sci.*(Paris), 203:1552-1554 (1936).
31. M. Czub, H.R. Braig, H. Diringer, Pathogenesis of scrapie, study of the temporal development of clinical symptons, of infectivity titres and scrapie-associated fibrils in brains of hamsters infected intraperitoneally, *J.Gen.Virol.*, 67:2005-2009 (1986).
32. M. Czub, H.R. Braig, H.Diringer, Replication of the scrapie agent in hamsters infected intracerebrally confirms the pathogenesis of amyloid-inducing virosis, *J.Gen.Virol.*, 69:1753-1756 (1988).
33. S. J. DeArmond, M.P. McKinley, R.A. Barry, M.B. Braunfeld, J.R. McColloch, S.B. Prusiner, Identification of prion amyloid filaments in scrapie-infected brain, *Cell*, 41:221-235 (1985).
34. A. G. Dickinson, H.Fraser, Scrapie, effect of Dh gene on the incubation period of extraneurally injected agent, *Heredity*, 29:91-93 (1972).
35. A. G. Dickinson, V.M.H. Meikle, Host genotype and agent effects in scrapie incubation, change in allelic interaction with different strains of agent, *Mol.Gen.Genet.*, 112:73-79 (1971).
36. A. G. Dickinson, V.M.H. Meikle, H.Fraser, Identification of a gene which controls the incubation period of some strains of scrapie in mice, *J.Comp.Pathol.*, 78:293-299 (1968).
37. A. G. Dickinson, D.M. Taylor, H. Fraser, Depression of polymorph counts by various scrapie agents, *Nature*, 248:510-511 (1974).
38. J. Diedrich, S. Wietgrefe, M. Zupancic, K. Staskus, E. Retzel, A.T. Haase, R. Race, The molecular pathogenesis in scrapie and Alzheimer's disease, *Microb.Pathog.*, 2:435-442 (1987).

39. H. Diringer, H. Gelderblom, H. Hilmert, M. Ozel, C. Edelbluth, R.H. Kimberlin, Scrapie infectivity, fibrils and low molecular weight protein, *Nature*, 306:471-478 (1983).
40. H. Diringer, H. Hilmert, D. Simon, E. Werner, B. Ehlers, Toward purification of the scrapie agent, Eur.J.Biochem., 134:555-560 (1983).
41. H. Diringer, H.C. Rahn, L. Bode, Antibodies to protein of scrapie-associated fibtilis, *Lancet*, ii:345 (1984)
42. B. Ehlers, H.Diringer, Dextrane sulphate 500 delays and prevents mouse scrapie by impairment of agent replication in spleen, *J.Gen.Virol.*, 65:1325-1330 (1984).
43. C. G. Farquhar, A.G. Dickinson, Prolongation of scrapie incubation period by an injection of dextrane sulphate 500 within the month before or after infection, *J.Gen.Virol.*, 67:463-473 (1986).
44. H. Fraser, The pathology of natural and experimental scrapie, *in*: 'Slow Virus Diseases of Animals and Man,' R.H. Kimberlin, ed., North Holland, Amsterdam, pp.267-305 (1976).
45. H. Fraser, A.G. Dickinson, The sequential development of the brain lesions of scrapie in three strains of mice, *J.Comp.Pathol.*, 78:301-311 (1968).
46. H. Fraser, A.G. Dickinson, Pathogenesis of scrapie in the mouse, the role of the spleen, *Nature*, 226:462-463 (1970).
47. H. Fraser, A.G. Dickinson, Studies of the lymphoreticular system in the pathogenesis of scrapie, the role of spleen and thymus, *J.Comp.Pathol.*, 88:563-573 (1978).
48. D. C. Gajdusek, Unconventional viruses and the origin and disappearance of kuru, *Science*, 197:943-960 (1977).
49. D. C. Gajdusek, Hypothesis: interference with axonal transport of neurofilament as a common pathogenetic mechanism in certain diseases of the central nervous system, *N.Engl.J.Med.*, 312:711-719 (1985).
50. D. C. Gajdusek, C.J. Gibbs, Jr., M. Alpers, Experimental transmission of a kuru-like syndrome to chimpanzees, *Nature*, 209:794-796 (1966).
51. D. C. Gajdusek, C.J. Gibbs, Jr., Subacute and chronic diseases caused by atypical infections with unconventional viruses in aberrant hosts, *in*: 'Perspective in Virology, vol.8,' M. Pollard, ed., Academic Press, New York, pp. 279-311 (1973).
52. D. C. Gajdusek, V. Zigas, Degenerative disease of the central nervous system in New Guinea, The endemic occurrence of 'kuru' in the native population, *N.Engl.J.Med.*, 257:974-978 (1957).
53. A. C. Gardiner, A.A. Marucci, Immunological responsiveness of scrapie infected mice, *J.Comp.Path.*, 79:233-235 (1969).
54. D. E. Garfin, D.P. Stites, J.D. Perlman, S.P. Cochran, S.B. Prusiner, Mitogen stimulation of splenocytes from mice infected with scrapie agent, *J.Infect.Dis.*, 138:396-400 (1978).
55. D. E. Garfin, D.P. Stites, L.A. Zitnik, S.B. Prusiner, Suppression of polyclonal B cell activation in scrapie infected C3H/HeJ mice, *J.Immunol.*, 120:1986-1990 (1978).
56. C. J. Gibbs Jr., D.C. Gajdusek, Isolation and characterization of the subacute spongiform virus encephalopathies of man: kuru and Creutzfeldt-Jakob disease, *J.Clin.Pathol.*, 25:84-96 (1972).
57. C. J. Gibbs Jr., D.C. Gajdusek, Experimental subacute spongiform virus encephalopathies in primates and other laboratory animals, *Science*, 182:67-68 (1973).
58. C. J. Gibbs Jr., D.C. Gajdusek, D.M. Asher, M.P. Alpers, E. Beck, P.M. Daniel, W.B. Matthews, Creutzfeldt-Jakob disease (subacute spongiform encephalopathy): transmission to the chimpanzee, *Science*, 161:388-389 (1968).
59. C. J. Gibbs Jr., D.C. Gajdusek, R. Latarjet, Unusual resistance to ionizing radiation of the viruses of kuru, Creutzfeldt-Jakob disease, and scrapie, *Proc.Natl.Acad.Sci.*, USA, 75:6268-6270 (1978).
60. W. S. Gordon, I.H. Pattison, The experimental production of scrapie in goats, *Vet.Rec.*, 69:1444 (1957).

61. P. D. Hart, M.R. Young, Interference with normal phagosome-lysosome fusion in macrophages using ingested yeast cells and suramin, *Nature*, 256:47 (1975).
62. M. S. Hirsch, Effect of antilymphocytic serum on host responses to infectious agents, *Fed.Proc.*, 29:169-170 (1970).
63. J. Hope, L.J.D. Morton, F. Farquhar, G. Multhaup, K. Beyreuther, R.H. Kimberlim: The major polypeptide of scrapie-associated fibrils (SAF) has the same size, charge distributions and N-terminal protein sequence has predicted for the normal brain protein (PrP). EMBRO J., 5:2591-2597 (1986).
64. J. Hope, G.Multhaup, L.J.D. Reekie, R.H. Kimberlin, K. Beyreuther, Molecular pathology of scrapie-associated fibril protein (PrP) in mouse brain affected by the ME7 strain of scrapie, *Eur.J.Biochem.*, 172:271-277 (1988).
65. N. Hunter, J. Hope, I. McConnell, A.G. Dickinson, Linkage of the scrapie-associated fibril protein (PrP) gene and sinc using congenic mice and restriction fragment length polymorphism analysis, *J.Gen.Virol.*, 69:2711-2716 (1987).
66. D. Karcher, B.S. Soler Federsppiel, F.D. Lowenthal, F. Frank, A. Lowenthal, Anti-neurofilament antibodies in blood of patients with neurological disease, *Acta Neuropathol.* (Berl.), 72:82-85 (1986).
67. K. C. Kasper, K. Bowman, D.P. Stites, S.B. Prusiner, Toward development of assays for scrapie-specific antibodies, *Adv.Exp.Med.Biol.*, 134:401-413 (1981).
68. K. C. Kasper, D.P. Stites, K.A. Bowman, H. Panitch, S.B. Prusiner, Immunological studies of scrapie infection, *J.Neuroimmunol.*, 3:187-201 (1982).
69. R. H. Kimberlin, P.G. Cunnington, Reduction of scrapie incubation time in mice and hamsters by a single injection of methanol extraction residue of BCG., *FEBS Microb.Lett.*, 3:169-172 (1978).
70. R. H. Kimberlin, C.A. Walker, Pathogenesis of mouse scrapie, dynamics of agent replication in spleen, spinal cord and brain after infection by different routes, *J.Comp.Pathol.*, 89:551-562 (1979).
71. R. H. Kimberlin, C.A. Walker, The antiviral compound HPA-23 can prevent scrapie when administered at the time of infection, *Arch.Virol.*, 78:9-18 (1983).
72. R. H. Kimberlin, C.A. Walker, Suppression of scrapie infection in mice by heteropolyanion 23, dextrane sulphate, and some other polyanions, *Antimicrob.Agents Chemother.*, 30:409-413 (1986).
73. D. T. Kingsbury, K.C. Kasper, D.P. Stites, J.D. Watson, R.N. Hogan, S.B. Prusiner, Genetic control of scrapie and Creutzfeldt-Jakob disease in mice, *J.Immunol.*, 131:491-496 (1983).
74. D. T. Kingsbury, D.A. Smeltzer, C.J. Gibbs Jr., D.C. Gajdusek, Evidence for normal cell-mediated immunity in scrapie-infected mice, *Infect. Immun.*, 32:1176-1180 (1981).
75. H. A. Kretzschmar, L.E. Stowring, D. Westway, W.H. Stubblebine, S.B. Prusiner, S.J. DeArmond, Molecular cloning of a human prion protein cDNA. *DNA*, 5:315-324 (1986).
76. Y. Kuroda, C.J. Gibbs Jr., H.L. Amyx, D.C. Gajdusek, Creutzfeldt-Jakob disease in mice, persistent viremia and preferential replication of virus in low-density lymphocytes, *Infect.Immun.*, 41:154-161 (1983).
77. A. Ladogana, P. Casaccia, S. Schmittinger, A. Iavarone, H.Y.G. Xi, C. Masullo, M. Pocchiari, Therapeutical approach in hamsters experimentally affected with scrapie: pathogenetic implications. Ageing Brain and Dementia, *Padua*, 22-24 September (1988).
78. G. C. Lavelle, L. Sturman, W.J. Hadlow, Isolation from mouse spleen of cell populations with high specific infectivity for scrapie virus, *Infect.Immun.*, 5:319-323 (1972).
79. Y. C. J. Liao, R.V. Lebo, G.A. Lawson, E.A. Smuckler, Human prion protein cDNA, molecular cloning, chromosomal mapping, and biological implications, *Science*, 233:364-367 (1986).

80. P. C. Licursi, P.A. Merz, G.S. Merz, R.I. Carp, Scrapie-induced changes in the percentage of polymorphonuclear neutrophils in mouse peripheral blood, *Infect.Immun.*, 6:370-376 (1972).
81. H. L. Lin, G. Medoff, G.S. Kobayashi, Effects of amphotericin B on macrophages and their precursor cells, *Antimicrob.Agents Chemother.*, 11:154-160 (1977).
82. C. Locht, B. Chesebro, R. Race, J.M. Keith, Molecular cloning and complete sequence of prion protein cDNA from mouse brain infected with the scrapie agent, *Proc.Natl.Acad.Sci.*, USA, 83:6372-6376 (1986).
83. G. Macchi, C. Masullo, M. Pocchiari, Le demenze trasmissibili, *Federazione Medica*, 38:1156-1160 (1985).
84. E. E. Manuelidis, Transmission of Cruetzfeldt-Jacob Disease from man to the guinea pig, *Science*, 190:571-572, (1975).
85. E. E. Manuelidis, Transmission of Creutzfeldt-Jakob disease with scrapie-like syndromes to mice, *Nature*, 271:778-779 (1978).
86. E. E. Manuelidis, J.N. Angelo, E.J. Gorgacz, L.Manuelidis, Transmission of Creutzfeldt-Jakob disease to Syrian hamsters, *Lancet*, i:479, (1977).
87. L. Manuelidis, T. Sklaviadis, E.E. Manuelidis, Evidence suggesting that PrP is not the infectious agent in Creutzfeldt-Jakob disease, *EMBO J.*, 6:341-347 (1987).
88. L. Manuelidis, S. Valley, E.E. Manuelidis, Specific proteins associated with Creutzfeldt-Jakob disease and scrapie share antigenic and carbohydrate determinants, *Proc.Natl.Acad.Sci.* USA, 82:4263-4267 (1985).
89. R. F. Marsh, Effect of vaccinia-activated macrophages on scrapie infection in hamsters, *in*: 'Hamster Immune Response in Infectious and Oncologic Diseases,' J.W. Streilein, D.A. Hart, J. Stein Streilein, W.R. Duncan, R.E. Billingham, eds., Plenum Press, New York, pp. 359-363 (1981).
90. R. F. Marsh, R.H. Kimberlin, Comparison of scrapie and transmissible mink encephalopathy in hamsters, II. Clinical signs, pathology and pathogenesis, *J.Infect.Dis.*, 131:104-110 (1975).
91. R. F. Marsh, J.M. Miller, R.P. Hanson, Transmissible mink encephalopathy, studies on the peripheral lymphocyte, *Infect.Immun.*, 7:352-355 (1973).
92. C. L. Masters, D.C. Gajdusek, C.J. Gibbs Jr., Creutzfeldt-Jakob disease virus isolation from the Gerstmann-Straussler syndrome, with an analysis of the various forms of amyloid plaque deposition in the virus-induced spongiform encephalopathies, *Brain*, 104:559-588 (1981).
93. C. L. Masters, G. Multhaup, G. Simms, J. Pottgiesser, R.N. Martins, K. Beyreuther, Neuronal origin of a cerebral amyloid: neurofibrillary tangles of Alzheimer's disease contain the same protein as the amyloid of plaque cores and blood vessels, *EMBO J.*, 4:2757-2763 (1985).
94. D. E. McFarlin, M.C. Raff, E. Simpson, S.H. Nehlsen, Scrapie in immunologically deficient mice, *Nature*, 233:336 (1971).
95. M. P. McKinley, D.C. Bolton, S.B. Prusiner, A protease-resistant protein is a structural component of scrapie prion, *Cell*, 35:57-62 (1983).
96. M. P. McKinley, M.B. Braunfeld, C.G. Bellinger, S.B. Prusiner, Molecular characteristics of prion rods purified from scrapie-infected hamster brains, *J.Infect.Dis.*, 154:110-120 (1986).
97. G. S. Merz, V. Schwenk, G. Schuller-Levis, S. Gruca, H.M. Wisniewski, Isolation and characterization of macrophages from scrapie-infected mouse brain, *Acta Neuropathol.(Berl.)* 72:240-247 (1987).
98. P. A. Merz, R.G. Rohwer, R. Kascsak, H.M. Wisniewski, R.A. Somerville, C.J. Gibbs Jr., D.C. Gajdusek, An infection specific particle from the unconventional slow virus diseases, *Science*, 225:437-440 (1984).
99. P. A. Merz, R.A. Somerville, H.M. Wisniewski, K. Iqbal, Abnormal fibrils from scrapie infected brain, *Acta Neuropathol.(Berl.)* 54:63-74 (1981).
100. R. K. Meyer, M.P. McKinley, K.A. Bowman, R.A. Barry, S.B. Prusiner, Separation and properties of cellular and scrapie prion proteins, *Proc.Natl.Acad.Sci.* USA, 83:2310-2314 (1986).
101. G. C. Millson, G.D. Hunter, R.H. Kimberlin, The physico-chemical nature of the scrapie agent, *in*: 'Slow Virus Diseases of Animals and Man,' R.H.

Kimberlin, ed., North Holland Publishing Company, Amsterdam, pp. 243-266 (1976).
102. S. Mohri, S. Handa, J.Tateishi, Lack of effect of thymus and spleen on the incubation period of Creutzfeldt-Jakob disease in mice, *J.Gen.Virol.*, 68:1187-1189 (1987).
103. G. Multhaup, H. Diringer, H. Hilmert, H. Prinz, J. Heukeshoven, K. Beyreuther, The protein component of scrapie-associated fibrils is a glycosylated low-molecular-weight protein, *EMBO J.*, 4:1495-1501 (1985).
104. B. Oesch, D. Westaway, M. Walchli, M.P. McKinley, S.B.H. Kent, R. Aebersold, R.A. Barry, P. Tempst, D.B. Teplow, L.E. Hood, S.B. Prusiner, C. Weissmann, A cellular gene encodes scrapie Prp 27-30 protein, *Cell*, 40:735-746 (1985).
105. H. B. Parry, Scrapie disease in sheep, D.R. Oppenheimer, ed., Academic Press, London, (1983).
106. M. Pocchiari, P. Casaccia, A. Iavarone, A. Ladogana, P. Mariotti, C. Masullo, S. Schmittinger, G. Macchi, Le encefalopatie spongiose subacute. *Quaderni di Neuropatologia*, 4:1-23 (1988).
107. M. Pocchiari, S. Schmittinger, A. Ladogana, C. Masullo, Effect of amphotericin B in intracerebral scrapie inoculated hamsters, *in*: 'Proc. II Symp. Int. sur les Virus non Conventionnels du Systeme Nerveux Central,' L.A. Court, D. Dormont, D. Kingsbury, eds., Abbay de Melleray, Moisdon la Riviere, in press (1989).
108. M. Pocchiari, S. Schmittinger, C. Masullo, Amphotericin B delays the incubation period of scrapie in intracerebrally inoculated hamsters, *J.Gen.Virol.*, 68:219-223 (1987).
109. S. B. Prusiner, D.C. Bolton, D.F. Groth, K.A. Bowman, S.P. Cochran, M.P. McKinley, Further purification and characterization of scrapie prions, *Biochemistry*, 21:6942-6950 (1982).
110. S. B. Prusiner, D.F. Groth, D.C. Bolton, S.B. Kent, L.E. Hood, Purification and structural studies of a major scrapie prion protein, *Cell*, 38:127-134 (1984).
111. S. B. Prusiner, M.P. McKinley, K.A. Bowman, D.C. Bolton, P.D. Bendheim, D.F. Groth, G.C. Glenner, Scrapie prions aggregate to form amyloid-like birefringent rods, *Cell*, 35:349-358 (1983).
112. N. K. Robakis, E.A. Devine-Gage, E.C. Jenkins, R.J. Kascsak, W.T. Brown, M.S. Krawczun, W.P. Silverman, Localization of a human gene homologous to the PrP gene of the p arm of chromosome 20 and detection of PrP-related antigens in normal human brain, *Biochem.Biophys.Res. Commun.*, 140:758-765 (1986).
113. N. K. Robakis, P.R. Sawh, G.C. Wolfe, R. Rubenstein, R.I. Carp, M.A. Innis, Isolation of a cDNA clone encoding the leader peptide of prion protein and expression of the homologous gene in various issues, *Proc.Natl. Acad.Sci.* USA, 83:6377-6381 (1986).
114. R. Rubenstein, R.J. Kascsak, P.A. Merz, M.C. Papini, R.I. Carp, N.K. Robakis, H.M. Wisniewski, Detection of scrapie-associated fibril (SAF) proteins using anti-SAF antibody in non-purified tissue preparations, *J.Gen.Virol.*, 67:671-681 (1986).
115. J. Sotelo, C.J. Gibbs Jr., D.C. Gajdusek, Autoantibodies against axonal neurofilaments in patients with kuru and Creutzfeldt-Jakob disease, *Science*, 210:190-193 (1980).
116. J. Sotelo, C.J. Gibbs Jr., D.C. Gajdusek, B.H. Toh, M. Wurth, Method for preparing cultures of central neurons: cytochemical and immunochemical studies, *Proc.Natl.Acad.Sci.* USA, 77:653-657 (1980).
117. R. S. Sparkes, M. Simon, V.H. Cohn, R.E.K. Fournier, J.Lem, I. Klisak, C. Heinzmann, C. Blatt, M. Lucero, T. Mohandas, S.J.DeArmond, D. Westway, S.B. Prusiner, L.P. Weiner, Assignment of the human and mouse prion protein genes to homologous chromosomes, *Proc.Natl.Acad.Sci.* USA, 83:7358-7362 (1986).

118. D. P. Stites, D.E. Garfin, S.B. Prusiner, The immunology of scrapie, *in*: 'Slow Transmissible Diseases of the Nervous System,' Vol. 2, S.B. Prusiner, W.J. Hadlow, eds., Academic Press, New York, pp. 211-221 (1979).
119. G. M. Stites, D. Barta, B.M. Olcott, W.F. Brown Jr., Serum and cerebrospinal fluid concentrations of immunoglobulin G in Suffolk sheep with scrapie. *Am.J.Vet.Res.*, 45: 1812-1813 (1984).
120. J. Tateishi, M.Ohta, N. Koga, Y. Sato, Y. Kuroiwa, Transmission of chronic spongiform encephalopathy with kuru plaque and leukomalacia of man to small rodents, *Ann.Neurol.*, 5:581-584 (1979).
121. B. H. Toh, C.J. Gibbs Jr., D.C. Gajdusek, J.Goudsmit, D. Dahl, The 200- and 150-kDa neurofilament proteins react with IgG autoantibodies from patients with kuru, Creutzfeldt-Jakob disease and other neurologic diseases, *Proc.Natl.Acad.Sci.* USA, 82:3485-3489 (1985).
122. B. H. Toh, C.J. Gibbs Jr., D.C. Gajdusek, D.D. Tuthill, D. Dahl, The 200-250-kDa neurofilament proteins react with IgG autoantibodies from chimpanzees with kuru or Creutzfeldt-Jakob disease; a 62-kDa neuro-filament-associated protein reacts with sera from sheep with natural scrapie, *Proc.Natl.Acad.Sci.* USA, 82:3894-3896 (1985).
123. G. A. H. Wells, A.C. Scott, C.T. Johnson, R.F. Gunning, R.D. Hancock, M. Jeffrey, M. Dawson, R. Bradley, A novel progressive spongiform encephalopathy in cattle, *Vet.Rec.*, 121:419-420 (1987).
124. E. S. Williams, S. Young, Chronic wasting disease of captive mule deer: a spongiform encephalopathy, *J.Wildlife Dis.*, 16:89-98 (1980).
125. M. Worthington, R. Clark, Lack of effect of immuno-suppression on scrapie infection, *J.Gen.Virol.*, 13:349-351 (1971).

INTRATHECAL IMMUNE RESPONSE IN HUMAN IMMUNODEFICIENCY VIRUS INFECTION

G.B. Zimatore, G. Angarano, I.L. Simone, S. Carbonara, C. Casalino, B. Coluccia, N. Panico, A. Rosato and P. Livrea

Institute of Neurology and Institute of Infectious Diseases, University of Bari, 70124 Bari, Italy

INTRODUCTION

Human immunodeficiency virus (HIV) is lymphotropic but also neurotropic and central nervous system (CNS) infection appears to be a biological feature of HIV.[21] Neurological disease occurs frequently in HIV infected patients and it can be the unique manifestation of the infection.[17] Recent reports suggest that biological and serological properties of some HIV subtypes are different in brain and in peripheral blood.[4]

Active immune surveillance and immune response in the CNS are mediated by interaction with the systemic immunity, and the systemic immunodepression may play a role in the pathogenesis of neurological diseases.[12] Therefore the HIV infection results either in neurological manifestations related to direct involvement of the nervous system or in diseases related to the immunodeficient state.

In an effort to clarify the natural history of HIV nervous system infection and to define the CSF profile of intrathecal immune response after HIV penetration into the nervous system, we have examined paired samples of CSF and serum from 80 HIV-seropositive patients, in various stages of disease, ranging from asymptomatic infection to AIDS.

MATERIALS AND METHODS

Paired samples of CSF and serum were obtained from 80 HIV-seropositive patients (11 females and 69 males, age 21-50 years). According to the risk factors of HIV infection in Italy,[1] 64 patients were intravenous drug abusers, four sexual partners of intravenous drug abusers, 10 homosexuals and two infected through blood transfusion. Twenty-six patients were classified as asymptomatic infection (ASI), 10 as persistent generalized lymphoadenopathy (PGL), 14 as acquired immunodeficiency syndrome related complex - (ARC), and 30 as AIDS.[2,3] Eighteen patients with neurological disease or with secondary CNS infections or neoplasms are included in the groups (AIDS-N). Twelve patients without neurological manifestations were considered separately (AIDS).

White cell count was performed on the fresh CSF samples (nv <5/μl). Glucose (enzymathic method), albumin and IgG (radial immunodiffusion) concentrations were carried out on CSF and serum. Normal values of CSF/serum glucose ratio were assumed to be higher than 0.55. The CSF/serum albumin

Table 1. Frequency of abnormal parameters in HIV-seropositive patients

	ASI	PGL	ARC	AIDS	AIDS-N
All CSF parameters normal	3 (12%)	1 (10%)	4 (28%)	0	1 (8%)
CSF white cells >5µl	11 (42%)	5 (50%)	2 (16%)	4 (33%)	1 (5%)
CSF/serum glucose <0.55	6 (23%)	0	4 (28%)	5 (41%)	10 (55%)
QA x 1000 >6.5	2 (7%)	1 (10%)	2 (14%)	2 (16%)	5 (28%)
CSF IgG Index >0.57	20 (77%)	8 (80%)	9 (64%)	9 (75%)	12 (66%)
CSF anti-HIV IgG synth.>3	11 (44%)	2 (20%)	2 (16%)	7 (58%)	8 (44%)
CSF oligoclonal bands	11 (52%)*	1 (12%)	1 (7%)	1 (8%)	1 (6%)
Serum HIV p24 antigen	9 (36%)	1 (10%)	11 (78%)†	6 (50%)†	14 (77%)†
CSF HIV p24 antigen	2 (8%)	0	2 (14%)	0	2 (16%)
Blood T helper <400/µl	13 (52%)	1 (10%)	14 (100%)#	10 (91%)#	11 (92%)#

Chi square: * p<0.002; † p<0.001; # p<0.001.

ratio x 1000 (QA) was used as a parameter of blood brain barrier (BBB) damage (nv <6.5) and the IgG Index as a measure of intra-BBB total IgG synthesis (nv <0.59). Abnormal CSF oligoclonal IgG fractions were detected by isoelectric focusing in thin layer polyacrylamide gel. HIV-specific IgG antibodies in CSF and serum were determined by Elisa (Behring), and the intrathecal anti-HIV IgG synthesis was calculated by CSF/serum antibody titre related to the blood brain barrier function[9,10] (nv <3). HIV p24 antigen was determined in CSF and serum by Elisa (Du Pont). Peripheral T helper lymphocyte count was performed by cytofluorimetry (Ortho Diagnostic System).

RESULTS

Table 1 summarizes the frequency of abnormal parameters in CSF and serum related to clinical diagnosis.

Normal CSF parameters were found with frequencies ranging between 0 to 28% irrespective of the diagnostic groups. An abnormal CSF leucocyte count was found with a lower percentage in AIDS-N patients (p<0.02), whereas the pleocytosis appeared more frequent in ASI and PGL patients. Low CSF/serum glucose ratio occurred without a significant relation to the stage of the disease; however a trend for a higher percentage seemed to exist in AIDS patients. Abnormalities in CSF/serum albumin ratio were found in every group, and their frequency increased from ASI to AIDS patients.

The intrathecal total and HIV-specific IgG synthesis appeared to be frequent findings, unrelated to the diagnostic groups and to the presence of neurological manifestations also. In the overall series, the intrathecal total and HIV-specific IgG synthesis were correlated (r= 0.62, p <0.01). Abnormal CSF IgG oligoclonal fractions were significantly more frequent in ASI patients (p<0.002). P24 antigen was found in CSF in few cases, whereas its presence in serum was significantly higher in ARC, AIDS and AIDS-N patients (p <0.0001). The same groups showed a decrease of peripheral T helper cell count (p<0.0001).

Patients subdivided according to blood T helper lymphocyte count (Table 2) showed a lack of intrathecal IgG oligoclonal fractions when T helper lymphocytes were lower than 100/µl. P24 antigen was found with higher frequency in serum and in CSF when T helper cells were lower than 400/µl and lower than 200/µl, respectively. The frequency of abnormal CSF/serum ratio of the albumin as well as of the glucose was unrelated to the blood T helper lymphocyte count. A decrease in blood T helper cells was accompanied by a decrease in CSF pleocytosis (p<0.006) and by a decreased frequency of total (p<0.04) and HIV-specific intrathecal IgG synthesis.

Table 2. Frequency of abnormal parameters in HIV-seropositive patients subdivided according to blood T helper count

T helper/µl	>400	<400 >200	<200 >400	<100
CSF white cells >5/µl	8/23 (34%)	9/15 (60%)	4/15 (26%)	1/19 (5%)#
CSF/serum glucose <0.55	4/23 (17%)	4/15 (26%)	5/15 (33%)	8/19 (42%)
QA x 1000 >6.5	2/23 (8%)	1/15 (6%)	3/15 (20%)	2/19 (10%)
CSF IgG Index >0.57	17/23 (74%)	13/15 (86%)	10/15 (66%)	11/19 (58%)*
CSF anti-HIV IgG synth >3	5/23 (22%)	9/15 (60%)	6/15 (40%)	6/19 (31%)
CSF oligoclonal bands	5/19 (26%)	6/14 (43%)	3/12 (25%)	0/18†
Serum HIV p24 antigen	2/23 (8%)§	8/15 (53%)	13/15 (86%)	13/19 (68%)
CSF HIV p24 antigen	0/23	0/15	3/15 (20%)	3/19 (16%)

Chi square: * $p<0.04$; † $p<0.03$; # $p<0.006$; § $p<0.001$.

Table 3. Intra-BBB total and HIV-specific IgG synthesis in HIV-seropositive patients subvided according to blood T helper count

T helper/µl	>400	<400 >200	<200 >400	<100
CSF IgG index	0.7 ± 0.24	0.95 ± 0.44*	0.76 ± 0.21	0.67 ± 1.8
CSF anti-HIV IgG synthesis	1.7 ± 1.7	7.25 ± 7.5†	3.70 ± 5	2.40 ± 1.7

ANOVA test: • $p<0.02$; † $p<0.003$.

Both total (ANOVA, $p<0.02$) and HIV-specific (ANOVA, $p<0.003$) IgG synthesis peaked when patients had blood T helper cells in the range 200-400//∝ (Table 3). The mean intrathecal HIV-specific IgG synthesis was significantly lower ($p<0.05$) in patients with T helper cell count higher than 400/µl compared to patients with T helper cell count lower than 400/µl (Table 4).

DISCUSSION

The intra-BBB HIV-specific IgG Synthesis[22,23] and the HIV isolation from CSF in ASI patients[5,23] indicate that the virus infects the CNS at an early stage. Our data confirm the presence of an intrathecal immune response in every phase of infection, irrespective of neurological manifestations.

According to other reports[19], the expression of p24 antigen in serum appears to be likely associated with a low number of blood T helper cells. Both antigenaemia[7,20] and the blood T helper cell count depletion[7,19,20] are significantly related to the later stages of the infection and they seem to mark disease progression. HIV p24 antigen in CSF is detectable in few cases and it is unrelated to individual diagnostic groups;[14] nevertheless it is worthwhile noting that the presence of HIV p24 antigen occurs only when blood T helper cells are lower than 200/µl.

Common CSF features are not frequent findings in CNS HIV infection. Abnormal values of albumin and glucose CSF/serum ratio are unusual and scattered in individual diagnostic groups. Nevertheless, both parameters seem to increase along with the progression of infection and the involvement of CNS[5,16] abnormal glucose but not albumin ratio shows a relationship with the blood T helper cell reduction. It is conceivable that BBB impairment is related to the duration of the infection. CSF leucocytes increase in the early stages of the infection, thereafter they subside, mainly in AIDS-N patients.[8] The lack of CSF

Table 4. Intra-BBB total and HIV-specific IgG synthesis in HIV-seropositive patients sub divided according to blood T helper count

T helper/µl	>400	<400
CSF IgG index	0.70 ± 0.24	0.78 ± 0.32
CSF anti-HIV IgG synthesis	1.70 ± 1.7*	4.22 ± 5.6

Student *t* test: * $p<0.05$.

cellular reaction during the infection progression results from the immunodepression and marks a poor prognosis; accordingly, it is significantly associated to blood T helper cell count lower than 100/µl.

The frequency of total intrathecal IgG synthesis is high in every diagnostic group, whereas the HIV-specific one appears to be less frequent. However, these parameters correlate each other. The HIV-specific immune response is only a fraction of the total intrathecal IgG production, which follows a polyclonal B cell activation.[22] The mechanism that induces the polyclonal B cell activation in both intrathecal and systemic immune system is at present unexplained and it appears as a finding of the immunological disorder.[15] Despite polyclonal hypergammaglobulinemia, the patients are refractory to antigenic stimuli and they are unable to develop specific antibody responses.[18] The intrathecal oligoclonal IgG fractions are detected with low frequency (14/63 patients), but, according to other reports,[9] this kind of immune response is significantly more common in ASI patients. The lack of oligoclonal fractions could reflect the impairment of B cell clone proliferation and differentiation in response to specific antigens.[6,13] Detection of oligoclonal IgG fractions could indicate a specific disease course or a stage of disease with preserved ability to produce an antibody response to viral antigens. Grimaldi et al.[11] supposed that the oligoclonal fractions are anti-p24-specific IgG which are lacking during the disease progression. Our data indicate that the oligoclonal IgG fractions are undetectable when T helper cell count is lower than 100/µl. The HIV cytopathic effect on T helper lymphocytes, combined with qualitative abnormalities, produces an impairment of immunological memory and a reduction of clonal expansion.

Patients subdivided according to blood T helper cell count show high frequency and high mean values of both total and HIV-specific intrathecal IgG synthesis when T helper cells are between 400-200/µl. In patients with T helper cell count higher than 400/µl, the total and the HIV-specific intrathecal IgG synthesis is detectable in 74% and 22% of cases, respectively. Accordingly, such patients show low values of HIV-specific, but not total, intrathecal IgG synthesis when compared to patients with T helper cells lower than 400/µl. In conclusion, when T helper cells are higher than 400/µl, a total intrathecal IgG synthesis is not always associated with specific anti-HIV response.

These findings suggest that, when peripheral T helper cells are normal, the virus is restricted in the brain and it escapes the intrathecal immune surveillance,[24] as indicated by a low HIV-specific response. Nevertheless, a polyclonal B cell activation and/or an alteration in the mechanisms controlling the IgG production occur during HIV latency phase. In the latency phase the viral RNA is present in T4 cells but it is not translated until they are immune activated. Activated cells have been recently supposed to express the viral antigen on their surface before viral production.[13] The substantial HIV immune response detected in patients with blood T helper cell count between 400 and 200/µl supports an antigen expression at the cell membrane preceding the viral release and the premature cell death. Longitudinal CSF studies may be an useful tool in assessing the natural history and the therapeutic response in CNS HIV infection.

REFERENCES

1. G. Angarano, G. Pastore, L. Monno, T. Santantonio, N. Luchena, O. Schiraldi, Rapid spread of HTLV-III infection among drug addicts in Italy, *Lancet* ii, 1302 (1985).
2. Centers for Disease Control, Classification system for Human T-Lymphotropic Virus type III/ Lymphadenopathy-Associated VIrus Infections, *MMWR*, 35:334-339 (1986).
3. Centers for Disease Control, Revision of the CDC surveillance case definition for acquired immunodeficiency syndrom, *MMWR*, 36:3-18 (1987).
4. C. Cheng-Mayer, J.A. Levy, Distinct biological and serological properties of Human Immunodeficiency Viruses from the brain, *Ann Neurol.*, 23(suppl):S58-S61 (1988).
5. F. Chiodi, A. Sönnerborg, J. Albert, H. Gaines, G. Norkrans, L. Hagberg, B. Asjö, O. Strannegard and EM Fenyö, Human Immunodeficiency Virus infection of the brain. I. Virus isolation and detection of HIV specific antibodies in the cerebrospinal fluid of patients with varying clinical conditions, *J.Neurol Sci.*, 85:245-257 (1988).
6. F. Chiodi, G. Norkrans, L. Hagberg, A. Sönnerborg, H. Gaines, S. Floland, EM Fenyö, E. Norrby and B. Vandvik, Human Immunodeficiency Virus infection of the brain II. Detection of intrathecally synthesized antibodies by enzyme linked immunosorbent assay and imprint immunofixation, *J.Neurol.Sci.*, 87:37-48 (1988).
7. F. de Wolf, J.M.A. Lange, J.T.M. Houweling, R.A. Coutinho, P.T. Schellekens, J. van der Noordaa, J. Goudsmit: Numbers of CD4+ cells and the levels of core antigens and of antibodies to the Human Immunodeficiency Virus as predictors of AIDS among seropositive homosexual men, *J.Infect Dis.*, 158:615-622, (1988).
8. I. Elovaara, M. Iivanainen, S.L. Valle, J. Suni, T. Tervo and J. Lahdevirta, CSF protein and cellular profiles in various stages of HIV infection related to neurological manifestation, *J.Neurol.Sci.*, 78:331-342 (1987).
9. J. Goudsmit, E.C. Wolters, M. Bakker, L. Smit, J. van der Noordaa, E.A.M. Hische, J.A. Tutuarima and van der Helm, Intrathecal synthesis of antibodies to HTLV-III in patients without AIDS or AIDS related complex, *Br.Med.J.*, 292:1231-1234 (1986).
10. J. Goudsmit, L.G. Epstein, D.A. Paul, H.J. van der Helm, G.J. Dawson, D.M. Asher, R. Yanagihara, A.V. Wolff, C.J. Gibbs jr. and D.C. Gajdusek, Intra-blood-brain barrier synthesis of human immunodeficiency virus antigen and antibody in humans and chimpanzees, *Proc.Natl.Acad.Sci.*, USA, 84:3876-3880 (1987).
11. L. M. E. Grimaldi, A. Castagna, R. Novati, P. Ronchi, R. Pristerà, A. Lazzarin, Applicaxione della tecnica dell'Isoelectic Focusing Antigen Overlay (IEF-O) alla caratterizzazione della risposta oligoclonale in liquor (LCR) di soggetti con infezione da HIV, in: 'Riassunti del II Convegno Nazionale AIDS e Sindromi Correlate,' OIC Medical Press, Milano, 60, (1988).
12. S. A. Houff, Neuroimmunology of Human Immunodeficiency Virus infection, in; AIDS and the nervous system, M.L. Rosemblum et al, eds., Raven Press, New York, 347-375 (1988).
13. R. Leonard, D. Zagury, I. Desportes, J. Bernard, J.F. Zagury and R.C. Gallo, Cytopathic effect of human immunodeficiency virus in T4 cells is linked to the last stage of virus infection, *Proc.Natl.Acad.Sci.*, USA, 85:3570-3574 (1988).
14. J. C. McArthur, B.A. Cohen, H. Farzedegan, D.R. Cornblath, O.A. Selnes, D. Ostrow, R.T. Johnson, J. Phair, and F. Polk: Cerebrospinal fluid abnormalities in homosexual men with and without neuropsychiatric findings, *Ann.Neurol.*, 23 (suppl):S34-S37, (1988).
15. H. Mizuma, S. Litwin and S. Zolla-Pazner, B-cell activation in HIV infection: relationship of spontaneous immunoglobulin secretion to various immunological parameters, *Clin.exp.Immunol.*, 71:410-416 (1988).
16. B. A. Navia, B.D. Jordan and R.W. Price, The AIDS Dementia Complex, I.Clinical features, *Ann Neurol.*, 19:517-524 (1986).

17. B. A. Navia, R.W. Price, The acquired immunodeficiency syndrome dementia complex as the presentig or sole manifestation of Human Immunodeficiency Virus infection, *Arch Neurol.*, 44:65-69 (1987).
18. S. G. Pahwa, M.T.J. Quilop, M. Lange, R.N. Pahwa & M.H. Grieco, Defective B-lymphocytes function in homosexual men in relation to the acquired immunodeficiency syndrome, *Ann.Int.Med.*, 101:757 (1984).
19. C. Pedersen, C.M. Nielsen, B.F. Vestergaard, J.Gerstoft, K. Krogsgaard, J.O. Nielsen, Temporal relation of antigenaemia and loss of antibodies to core antigens to development of clinical disease in HIV infection, *Br.Med.J.* 295:567-569 (1987).
20. B. F. Polk, R. Fox, R. Brookmeyer, S. Kanchanaraska, R. Kaslow, B. Visscher, C. Rinaldo and J. Phair, Predictors of the acquired immunodeficiency syndrome developing in a cohort of seropositive homosexual men, *N.Engl.J.Med.*, 316:61-66 (1987).
21. R. W. Price, J. Sidtis, M. Rosenblum, The AIDS Dementia Complex: some current questions, *Ann.Neurol*, 23(suppl): S27-S33, (1988).
22. L. Resnick, F. diMarzo-Veronese, J.Schupbach, W.W. Tourtellotte, D.D. Ho, F. Muller, P. Shapshak, M. Vogt, J.E. Groopman, P.D. Markham and R.C. Gallo, Intra-blood-brain barrier synthesis of HTLV-III-specific IgG in patients with neurologic symptoms associated with AIDS or AIDS-Related Complex, *N.Engl.J.Med.*, 313:1498-1504 (1985).
23. L. Resnick, J.R. Berger, P.Shapshak and W.W. Tourtellotte, Early penetration of the blood-brain-barrier by HIV, *Neurology*, 38:9-14 (1988).
24. S. Roy and M.A. Wainberg, Role of the Mononuclear Phagocyte System in the development of Acquired Immunodeficiency Syndrome (AIDS). *J.Leuk Biol.*, 43:91-97 (1988).

COMPARTMENTALIZATION OF B CELL RESPONSE TO CSF IN LYME DISEASE WITH NEUROLOGICAL MANIFESTATIONS

Shahid Baig, Tomas Olsson and Hans Link

Department of Neurology, Karolinska Institutet, Huddinge University Hospital, S-141 86 Huddinge Stockholm, Sweden

ABSTRACT

The *Borrelia burgdorferi*-specific B cell response in CSF and peripheral blood (PB) from patients with Lyme disease and neurological manifestations was studied with a nitrocellulose immunospot assay, enabling enumeration of cells secreting anti-*Borrelia* IgG, IgA and IGM antibodies. Such cells were found in CSF from most patients with neuroborreliosis, at mean values amounting to 32%, 40% and 34%, respectively, of IgG, IgA and IgM secreting cells in CSF. Anti-*Borrelia* antibody producing cells were only occasionally demonstrable in PB and then at very low numbers, reflecting a specific B cell response which is highly compartmentalized to CSF-CNS. Evaluation of B cell response at cellular level yields a different and more authentic picture of humoral immunity in comparison with conventional serology.

INTRODUCTION

Neurological manifestations in the form of meningo-radiculitis, meningitis or involvement of one or more cranial nerves may occur in Lyme disease[1]. Less frequently, clinical evidence of parenchymal CNS lesions may be present (for review see reference 2). CSF findings characteristically consist of mononuclear pleocytosis and blood-brain barrier (BBB) damage which both may be pronounced, evidence of intra-BBB synthesis of IgG, IgA and especially of IgM as reflected by, eg. elevated index values for these Ig, and oligoclonal IgG bands.[1-3]. A history of tick-bite and of erythema migrans may guide the diagnosis which is usually verified by demonstration of IgG and IgM antibodies against the etiologic spirochete *B.burgdorferi* in serum and particularly in CSF.[5]

Since levels of specific antibodies present in free form in body fluids, especially in a compartment such as CSF, may be influenced by a variety of factors including binding to target structures and catabolism, we have addressed the question whether enumeration of cells secreting specific antibodies of different isotypes might yield information beyond that obtained by conventional serology.[6,7] When studying patients with Lyme disease with neurological manifestations, we have now found that this disease during its acute and subacute stages is regularly accompanied by presence of *B. burgdorferi* antibody secreting cells in CSF but rarely in peripheral blood, thus reflecting a specific B cell response which is highly sequestrated to CSF-CNS.

MATERIALS AND METHODS

Paired specimens of CSF and peripheral blood were obtained from 15 consecutive patients with neurological signs and symptoms indicative of Lyme disease with neurological manifestations, and in whom routine serology for *B.burgdorferi* was unequivocally positive. In 12 of the patients, CSF and blood specimens were obtained within 45 days after onset of neurological symptoms, while longer time intervals had elapsed in the remaining three patients. Most patients had a pronounced mononuclear pleocytosis in CSF, and only one had a CSF cell count which was borderline. Elevated CSF/plasma albumin ratio reflecting BBB damage[8] was found in nine of fourteen patients examined. Agarose isoelectric focusing (AIF) of unconcentrated CSF and diluted plasma followed by protein transfer to nitrocellulose membrane and immunostaining[9] revealed oligoclonal IgG bands selectively in CSF in 12 patients indicating intra-BBB IgG synthesis, while one patient had oligoclonal bands in CSF and plasma simultaneously and the remaining two patients were negative for oligoclonal bands. *Borrelia burgdorferi* serology was positive in serum and CSF in 12 patients and in CSF exclusively in the remaining three (Table 1).

Borrelia burgdorferi strain Aca-1 isolated from the skin of a Swedish patient with acrodermatitis chronica atrophicans[10] was prepared as described[11] and used as antigen in immunospot assay. Immunoreactivity of the preparation was tested by ELISA,[12] employing sera previously known to be positive and negative for antibodies against *B. burgdorferi*. A dilution of the antigen preparation (generally amounting to 1 µg of protein/ml as determined by UV spectrophotometry) giving absorbance values which clearly discriminated these sera, was used for coating in the immunospot assay.

Samples of CSF (20 ml) were taken. After cell counting and centrifugation, cells (CSF-L) were resuspended in tissue culture medium (TCM) and recentrifuged, followed by redilution to cell concentration of 4-50 x 10^4 cells/ml. Peripheral blood was taken simultaneously, and lymphocytes (PBL) were separated, washed, rediluted in TCM, counted and adjusted to 10^6 cells/ml.

A solid-phase enzyme-linked immunospot assay[13,14] employing microtitre plates with 96 wells and nitrocellulose bottoms was used.[15]. Coating was carried out over night at 4°C with 100 µl aliquots per well of *B.burgdorferi* in solution for enumeration of antibody producing cells, or with 100 µl of diluted affinity purified goat anti-human IgG, IgA and IgM, heavy chain specific for enumeration of total numbers of IgG, IgA and IgM producing cells. Optimal antigen concentrations in coating solutions were defined in preliminary experiments. Coating solutions were removed by suction, the plates were washed with PBS, and 100 µl aliquots containing 10^5 PBL or 4-50 x 10^3 CSF-L were applied into individual wells. After incubation overnight, wells were emptied and washed. Diluted high affinity purified biotinylated goat anti-human IgG, IgA or IgM (100 µl) (Sigma) was added to appropriate wells followed by washing and incubation with diluted avidin-biotin peroxidase complex. After washing, plates were stained with 3-amino-9-ethylcarbazole (Sigma) and H_2O_2 as substrate,[16] washed and dried. Formed immunospots were counted in a dissection microscope at a magnification of x 25. Values obtained were standardized to number of spots per 10^4 cultured cells.

RESULTS

Numbers of cells secreting anti-*Borrelia* IgG, IgA and IgM antibodies, and total numbers of IgG, IgA and IgM producing cells per 10^4 CSF-L or PBL are presented in Table 1 and Fig. 1 Antibody secreting cells were found in CSF in all 15 patients except in No. 15 whose symptoms probably started 1.5 years before

Table 1. Numbers of cells per 10^4 mononuclear cells in CSF and blood producing IgG, IgA and IgM antibodies against B.burgdorferi, related to total numbers of IgG, IgA and IgM producing cells, in patients with Lyme disease with neurological manifestations.

Patient	IgG		IgA		IgM		Borrelia serology	
No.	CSF	PB	CSF	PB	CSF	PB	CSF	Serum
1	18/72	1/2	2/6	0/3	4/3	0/1	+	-
2	18/25	0/1	0/11	0/1	0/15	0/0	+	-
3	0/40	1/3	0/3	0/6	13/9	1/2	+ *	+ *
4	37/14	0/6	6/45	0/9	29/88	0/5	+	-
5	2/14	0/3	2/3	0/4	1/9	0/3	+	+
6	3/128	0/12	7/7	0/3	7/80	0/3	+	+
7	12/64	0/2	0/20	0/10	3/8	0/2	+	+
8	19/50	0/5	0/25	0/10	0/20	0/1	+	+
9	16/81	0/3	6/6	0/6	2/6	0/4	+	+
10	3/28	0/6	2/26	0/12	2/7	0/4	+	-
11	30/11	0/4	19/8	0/1	5/nd	0/2	+	+
12	32/42	0/1	nd/nd	nd/3	nd/nd	nd/1	+	+
13	57/85	0/1	26/20	0/7	6/10	0/1	+	+
14	3/28	0/2	nd/nd	0/4	nd/nd	0/1	+	+
15	0/5	0/2	0/3	0/5	0/1	0/2	+	+

* Serology positive for IgM antibodies only. nd = Not done.

examination. Intra-BBB presence of cells secreting antibodies of all three isotypes were found in eight of the patients, while two had IgG and IgM antibody secreting cells, and four had only IgG antibody secreting cells. One patient had only IgM antibody secreting cells in CSF, and in this patient (No.3) serology was positive for anti-*Borrelia* IgM antibodies exclusively.

The proportion of cells secreting anti-*Borrelia* IgG antibodies demonstrable in CSF constituted 32% (range 0-100%) of the total number of IgG producing cells. Figures for IgA antibody secreting cells were 40% (range 0-100%) and for IgM 34% (range 0-100%) (Fig. 2).

Interestingly, only two of the patients had minimal numbers of cells secreting antibodies against *B. burgdorferi* in peripheral blood, while the remaining patients were negative. This means that the specific B cell response which we have registered in neuroborreliosis is highly sequestrated to CSF-CNS.

DISCUSSION

The possibility of defining the number of cells secreting specific antibodies in body fluids introduces a new dimension in the evaluation of the B cell response, by passing some of the drawbacks which are inherent to conventional serological determinations of corresponding antibodies present in free form in body fluids since, for example, antibody binding to target structures and catabolism may make the detection of free antibodies impossible or unpredictable[7]. The presently used nitrocellulose immunospot assay allows enumeration of cells producing specific antibodies of different isotypes and the total number of IgG, IgA and IgM producing cells in parallel. Since the systems used for detection of specific antibody and Ig secretion probably have different sensitivity, caution must be taken when evaluating the proportion of antibody secreting cells among total Ig secreting cells of a certain isotype. The immunospot assay can safely be used even when few cells are available, the minimum number

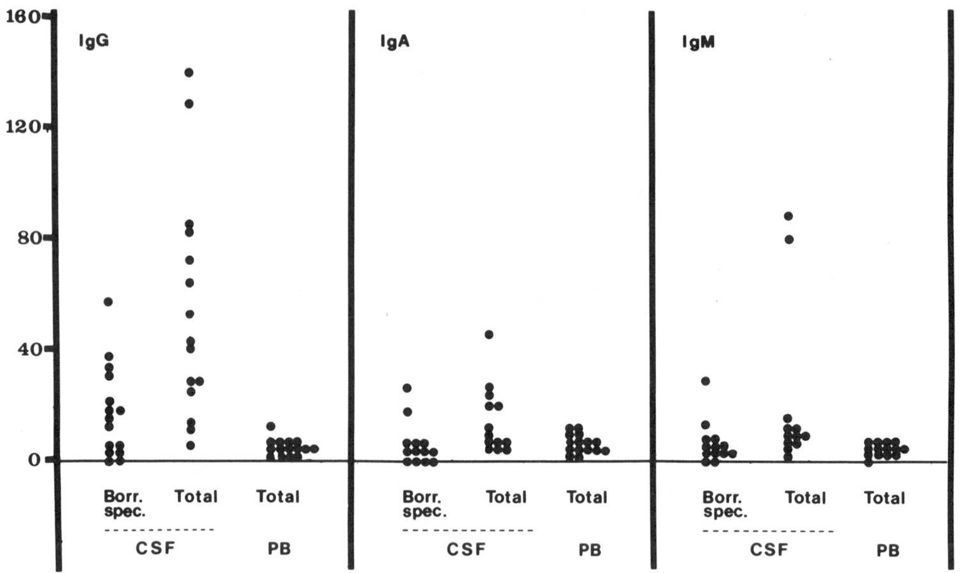

Fig. 1. Number of immunospots per 10^4 cultivated cells recovered from the cerebrospinal fluid (CSF) and peripheral blood (PB). Anti-*B. burgdorferi* antibody secreting (*Borrelia* sp) and total number of immunoglobulin secreting (total) cells of the different isotypes are shown.

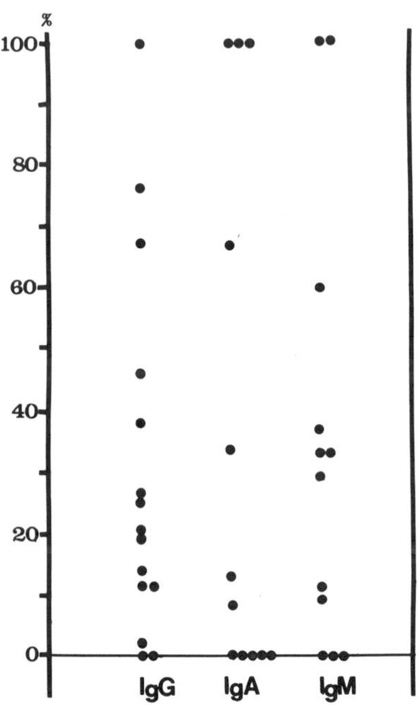

Fig. 2. The Number of demonstrable anti-*B. burgdorferi* secreting cells in per cent of total number of immunoglobulin secreting cells of the different isotypes in neuroborreliosis.

of cells necessary being 4000 per well to enable safe calculations. Whether the results obtained with the immunospot assay reflect the situation *in vivo* cannot be settled, and we cannot exclude the possibility that factors involved in sampling and short-term cultivation may influence the results. On the other hand, our data for IgG, IgA and IgM producing cells in peripheral blood from healthy controls obtained with the immunospot assay are similar to those previously reported with an indirect hemolytic protein A plaque assay, and results from this assay are generally accepted as reflecting the *in vivo* situation.

When assessing the antibody response against *B. burgdorferi* at the cellular level, the question also arises whether the formed immunospots are the results of active antibody secretion or represent shedding of cytophilic antibodies. Since immunospot formation can be suppressed by inhibition of secretion with monesin as well as of protein synthesis with cycloheximide, and kinetic studies of spot formation have revealed increasing size of immunospots with increasing incubation times (data not shown), we consider that the immunospots which we have enumerated are the result of secretion. Non-specific binding of Igs in the immunospot assay is unlikely since cells secreting antibodies against *B. burdorferi* were only occasionally demonstrated in peripheral blood, and absent in CSF and peripheral blood from patients with aseptic meningoencephalitis and non-inflammatory neurological diseases despite high numbers of cells secreting Igs (data not shown).

It is well established that Lyme disease with neurological manifestations is frequently accompanied by a BBB damage as well as evidence for intra-BBB inflammation, the latter being reflected by mononuclear pleocytosis, oligoclonal IgG bands and increased index values for IgG, IgA and especially IgM.[3,4,17]. On the other hand, calculations of these index values have been shown to be less reliable in presence of BBB damage, particularly if pronounced as it may occur in neuroborreliosis.[18] Similar errors may be inherent to calculation of a 'spirochetal CSF titre index' equal to (ELISA titre in CSF/ELISA titre in serum):(CSF albumin/serum albumin) which has been reported to be increased for IgG and IgM antibodies in neuroborreliosis.[5]

Our finding that neuroborreliosis is regularly accompanied by presence of cells in CSF secreting IgG, IgA and/or IgM antibodies against *B.burgdorferi* provides proof that an intra-BBB specific antibody response regularly occurs in this disease and that the previously described elevated values for IgG, IgA and especially IgM in CSF are not exclusively a result of BBB damage. Furthermore, we can draw the conclusion that the specific antibody response in neuroborreliosis is compartmentalized to CSF-CNS. The *B.burgdorferi* antibodies present in serum thus obviously do not originate from circulating plasma cells. One must therefore envisage specific antibody production in peripheral lymphoid organs. It can then only be speculated upon which mechanisms are responsible for recruitment into CSF and CNS of plasma cells secreting *B.burgdorferi* antibodies. For T cells, it has been suggested that they pass into the CNS if they are activated and irrespective of specificity, while further pathophysiological events occur when the T cells then recognize their specific antigen[19]. If similar mechanisms apply to B cells in neuroborrelisois, a random passage into CSF-CNS of B cells- - which then probably are *B. burgdorferi* specific at a rather high frequency - leads to contact with specific antigen, in this case the spirochete *B. burgdorferi*. A consequence would be further proliferation and maturation into plasma cells secreting specific antibodies. This process would require local T cell help. Indeed, *B. burgdorferi* specific T cells have been demonstrated in neuroborreliosis.[20]

Since not all immunoglobulin producing cells found in the CSF in neuroborreliosis have specificity for the causative organism, function of remaining cells may be questioned. Firstly, all cells might still be *B. burgdorferi* specific, but the cells hitherto unidentified regarding antibody specificity may be directed against *B. burgdorferi* antigens not accessible for binding in our assay. Secondly, the cells may in fact be directed against other epitopes not related to *B. burgdorferi*, either as result of non-specific recruitment or because of specific immune response against, eg, nervous tissue components. Intra-BBB production of antibodies against myelin has been reported in neuroborreliosis,[21] and we have also preliminary evidence when using the immunospot assay that cells are present in the CSF producing antibodies against myelin as well as myelin basic protein (data not shown). Whether such antibodies have relevance for pathogenesis of neurological manifestations in neuroborreliosis is an open question. Thirdly, the cells may be involved in synthesis of antiidiotypic antibodies.

Regarding biological role of locally produced antibodies, they may have antimicrobial function through either complement mediated lysis or opsonization for macrophage attack. Another potentially important role is the capacity of B cells to act as antigen presenting cells for T cells, due to expression of class II transplantation antigen and expression of surface receptor for antigen in form of specific immunoglobulin, thereby enabling concentration of antigen occurring in low amounts.[22] This may be of special relevance in *B. burgdorferi* infection where the spirochete is known to be only sparsely distributed *in vivo*.

ACKNOWLEDGEMENTS

This study was supported in part by the Swedish Medical Research Council (projects No. 3381 and 7488). The qualified secretarial help by Ms Yvonne Nilsson is highly acknowledged.

REFERENCES

1. A. R. Pachner and A.C. Steere, The triad of neurologic manifestations of Lyme disease: meningitis, cranial neuritis and radiculoneuritis, *Neurology*, 35:47 (1985).
2. S. Fredrikson and H. Link, CNS-borreliosis selectively affecting central motor neurons, *Acta Neurol.Scand.*, 78:181 (1988).
3. K. Felgenhauer, Differentiation of the humoral immune response in inflammatory diseases of the central nervous system, *J.Neurol.*,228:223 (1982).
4. A. Henriksson, H. Link, M. Cruz and G. Stiernstedt, Immunoglobulin abnormalities in cerebrospinal fluid and blood over the course of lymphocytic meningoradiculitis (Bannwarth's syndrome), *Ann.Neurol.*, 20:337 (1986).
5. G. Stiernstedt, M. Granström, B, Gederstedt and B. Sköldenberg, Diagnosis of spirochetal meningitis by enzyme-linked immunosorbent assay and indirect immunofluorescence assay in serum and cerebrospinal fluid, *J.Clin.Microbiol.*, 21:819 (1985).
6. H. Link, CSF IgG and its congeners, *in*: 'Advances in CSF Protein Research and Diagnosis', E.J. Thompson, ed., MTP Press Ltd., Lancaster (1987).
7. H. Link, S. Kam-Hansen and A. Henriksson, Immunoglobulins, New approaches for their evaluation in multiple sclerosis, *in*: 'Cellular and Humoral Immunological Components of Cerebrospinal Fluid in Multiple Sclerosis,' A. Lowenthal and J. Raus, eds., Plenum Press, New York/London, pp.175-185 (1987).
8. G. Tibbling, H. Link and S. Öhman, Principles of albumin and IgG analysis in neurological disorders, I. Establishment of reference values, *Scand.J.Invest.*, 35:385 (1977).
9. T. Olsson, V. Kostulas and H. Link, Improved detection of oligoclonal IgG in cerebrospinal fluid by agarose isoelectric focusing, double antibody peroxidase and avidin-biotin amplification, *Clin.Chem.*, 30:1246 (1984).
10. E. Åsbrink, B. Hederstedt and A. Hovmark, The spirochetal etiology of acrodermatitis chronica atrophicans Herxheimer, *Acta Derm.Venerol.*, 64:506 (1984).

11. K. Hansen, P. Hindersson and N. Strandberg-Pedersen, Measurement of antibodies to the Borrelia burgdorferi Flagellum improves sero-diagnosis in Lyme disease, *J.Clin.Microbiol.*, 26:338 (1988).
12. E. Craft, R.L. Grodzicki and A.C. Steeere, Antibody response in Lyme disease: Evaluation of diagnostic tests, *J.Infect.Dis.*, 149:789 (1984).
13. C. C. Czerkinsky, L.A. Nilsson, H. Nygren et al., A solid-phase enzyme-linked immunospot (ELISPOT) assay for enumeration of specific antibody-secreting cells, *J.Immunol.Meth.*, 65:109 (1983).
14. J. D. Sedgweick and P.G. Holt, A solid-phase immunoenzymatic technique for the emuneration of specific antibody secreting cells, *J.Immunol.Meth*, 57:301 (1983).
15. S. A. Moller and C.A.R. Borrebaeck, A filter immunoplaque assay for the detection of antibody-secreting cells in vitro, *J.Immunol.Meth.* 79:195 (1985).
16. L. S. Kaplow, Substitute for benzidine in myeloperoxidase stains, *Am.J.Clin. Pathol.*, 63:451 (1975).
17. C. J. M. A. Sindic, G. Depré, G. Bigaignon, P.F. Hella and C. Laterre, Lymphocytic meningoradiculitis and encephalomyelitis due to Borrelia burgdorferi: a clinical and serological study of 18 cases, *J.Neurol. Neurosurg.Psychiat.*, 50:1565 (1987).
18. A. K. Lefvert and H. Link, IgG production within the central nervous system: A critical review of proposed formulae, *Ann.Neurol.*, 17:13 (1985).
19. H. Wekerle, C. Linington, H. Lassmann and R. Meyermann, Cellular immune reactivity within the CNS, *TINS* 9:271 (1986).
20. A. R. Pachner, A.C. Steere, L.H. Sigal and C.J. Johnson, Antigen-specific proliferation of CSF lymphocytes in Lyme disease, *Neurology*, 35:1642 (1985).
21. G. Suchanek, W. Kristoferitsch, G. Stanek and H. Bernheimer, Anti-myelin antibodies in cerebrospinal fluid and serum of patients with meningopolyneuritis Garin-Bujadoux-Bannwarth and other neurological diseases, *Zbl.Bakt.Hyg.*, A263:160 (1986).
22. A. Lanzavecchia, Antigen uptake and accumulation in antigen-specific B cells, *Immunol.Rev.*, 99:39 (1987).

AUTHOR INDEX

SUBJECT INDEX